Eat
Clean Up

YOUR PERSONAL JOURNEY TO A HEALTHY LIFE

MANJARI CHANDRA

L!FE

Published by

FiNGERPRINT! LiFE

An imprint of Prakash Books India Pvt. Ltd.

113/A, Darya Ganj, New Delhi-110 002,
Tel: (011) 2324 7062 – 65, Fax: (011) 2324 6975
Email: info@prakashbooks.com/sales@prakashbooks.com

facebook www.facebook.com/fingerprintpublishing
twitter www.twitter.com/FingerprintP
www.fingerprintpublishing.com

ISBN: 978 93 9018 382 1

Processed & printed in India

This book is dedicated to my parents
who have guided me through the crests and troughs of my life.
I would also like to dedicate this book to my patients, who have
conquered their diseases by sheer grit and discipline and the
choices of healthier lifestyles and nourishing food.

TESTIMONIALS

"My world had come to a standstill when I was diagnosed with non-Hodgkin's lymphoma four years ago. After a series of those painful sessions of radio and chemotherapy, I was finally nurturing hope when the PET scan didn't show any trace of cancerous cells. But, this happiness was short-lived as the follow-up scan after a couple of years showed that the tumours were again increasing in size. I was 43 and I felt as if it's the end. And then, I happened to meet Manjari who made me believe that even cancer can be managed through right nutrition. She immediately put me on a protocol of Fasting Mimicking Diet (FMD). I ate as per what, when, and how much she told me. I also followed her advice on physical activity. And now, I am happy to tell you that I am feeling better both physically and emotionally and the cancer seems to be going in remission."

Kavish Chandola, 43, Male

"A disease condition called autoimmune thyroid disorder and a bulky frame (BMI of 34) would have pushed me into depression if Manjari hadn't come to my rescue. Since medicines were of no use, she advised me to eat right and make healthy lifestyle changes in my life. She explained to me that the auto immunity required lifestyle correction and nutritional intervention, as medication would not be effective in my disease state. In no time, home-cooked fresh and nutritious food became my staple. I also followed her advice on doing regular exercises, having a good night's sleep, and practicing yoga and meditation. It's been around 18 months and I have already lost 24 kgs and am free of any pills or medications to manage my thyroid hormones."

Bhavna Sikri, 47, Female

"I have been facing gut issues like acid reflux, bloating, irregular bowel movement, stomach pain and loss of appetite for a long time now. At the age of 20, when my friends could eat anything, I was always carrying antacids, antibiotics, and painkillers with me. The condition aggravated as I moved to

London for higher studies. I also started to face skin problems like acne and hair fall. One of my friends recommended me to Manjari. I consulted her and after hearing me patiently she advised me an elimination diet. She helped me identify food allergens that were troubling me and suggested anti-inflammatory foods for gut healing. I must say these six months of consultation with Manjari have helped me a lot with my pain and acidity. I am no more dependent on drugs for relief. My quality of life has improved a lot now and I have regained my healthy skin and hair back."

Shraddha Banga, 20, Female

"We Kashmiris are very fond of eating, especially red meat and rice cooked with a lot of spices and fat. But, now at 60, the aftermath of unhealthy lifestyle reflects on my health. Hypertension, high cholesterol, and fluctuating BP were affecting my wellbeing. I was popping tens of pills every day. Frustrated by high amounts of medication, I sought Manjari's help, who recommended me a detox plan and oxygen therapy to eliminate toxic heavy metals from the body. Then she gave me a strict nutritional plan integrated with light exercising and brisk walking. After a few months of treatment I felt my belly and weight reducing. My cholesterol levels and blood pressure are also stable, all thanks to Manjari."

Azhar Sherwani, 60, Male

"Money can't buy health and happiness; nobody can understand this better than me. I am a 50-year-old wife of a jewellery tycoon. I had all the luxuries at my disposal, except for the moments of happiness. Except for me, everybody in my family was busy with their lives. I don't know when this loneliness translated into mental health problems. I was restricted to the walls of my house, mostly eating, which resulted in weight gain. Depression had grown on me severely by the time I met Manjari. She talked to me at length. I felt relaxed as I finally found someone who understood me. On her insistence, I started seeing a cognitive behaviour therapist. In addition, she suggested me a healthy diet plan and a fitness regimen. Within 4-5 months, I started feeling good about myself. Now, I go for walks, meet people, and partake in each other's joys. I have also lost weight and have started to see a life in a positive way. Thanks to Manjari for restoring hope in my life."

Meera Bhatia, 50, Female

FOREWORD

There has been a drastic rise in the incidence of non-alcoholic fatty liver diseases, liver disorders, gastrointestinal conditions such as IBS, GERD, and acid reflux, leading all the way to upper GI and colorectal cancer, and other related diseases over the past decade. A large part of these diseases can be attributed to unhealthy eating habits coupled with high stress and poor lifestyle.

While the recent advancements in the field of medicine have brought about significant improvement in the treatment outcomes of diseases associated with poor nutrition, preventing such problems in the first place can work wonders in minimizing the disease burden. The gut being the second brain of the body needs to be treated well with good and nutritious food. When it comes to liver and gut health in particular, heavy alcohol consumption, risk factors for Hepatitis C, having diabetes and hypertension are the major contributors.

Diabetes alone can increase one's risk of developing metabolic syndrome multifold. Therefore, it is important to make lifestyle adjustments if you have or are prone to diabetes. Right nutrition integrated with moderate physical activity can go a long way in managing diabetes as well as other problems like heart disease, hormonal imbalances, and recovery from cancer. That's where Manjari Chandra has been making a commendable contribution by highlighting the role of nutrition in the prevention and treatment of a number of health problems.

I am quite impressed with her idea of healthy eating and nutrition for health and wellness. A firm believer in the old adage 'let food be thy medicine', she has always emphasized on the need of eating home-cooked fresh and natural foods. She has this amazing convincing power that makes her patients believe in her advice. And needless to say they end up benefiting from her expertise.

Eat Up, Clean Up is a book on healing. It is loaded with heaps of useful lessons on what, when, and how to eat. It will show you how you have forgotten to eat right. It will prove to you how a few yards of morning walk is better than your never-ending rat race. And finally, it will tell you how some fun moments in your living room and an hour in your kitchen can boost your health and well-being.

Happy Wellness.

Padma Shri Dr Saumitra Rawat

CONTENTS

CHAPTER ONE

Nutrition: From a Need to a Trade

Food has become our confidante in happiness, sadness, and fashionably so in fitness. While fitness may have gained more screen footage in recent times, we've lost the path that brings us good health. With newer and stranger diseases on the rise, this is the time to take a step back and reflect on what we pump into our body every single day.

You can argue that with technological advancement, the medical space has found solutions to unknown ailments. Unlike in the past we now have treatments available for cancer, diabetes, tuberculosis, and even the common cold. So why bother monitoring your diet to the T? After all, life was meant to be lived, not fretted over. Well, herein lies the problem. The pharmaceutical industry has instilled in our minds the belief that because we dominate the food chain, we are an immortal species. A couple of pills over a couple of weeks and all is well. But, what about the extra economic burden that comes in tow as medical costs and of course not to forget the additional hazards of preferring medicine over healthy food, which bypasses the age-old wisdom of letting 'thy food be thy medicine'?

Let's talk about the economic burden first. According to a study published in the *BMJ*, 'around 80% of populations are reportedly spending out-of-pocket (OOP) while seeking treatment, during 2011–2012. The proportion of the population reporting any OOP payments has increased sharply from about 60% during 1993–1994 to 80% in 2011–2012.'

Talking about the health hazards now, isn't taking medicines for anything and everything compromising the natural healing ability or simply the immunity of our body? What this means is that we are making our bodies more and more dependent on pills and medication. It is no wonder then that Crocin and Cocaine both go by the name of drugs. After all, both can lead to serious addiction.

Overall, from 'eating for hunger' to 'eating for taste', our food preferences have undergone a shift that we can never be apologetic enough for. Don't animals have an advantage over humans when it comes to food? Let's face the reality!

What is Nutrition?

Most of us tend to view nutrition through green-coloured lenses—a lifestyle that symbolizes all greens and zero flavours. A dietary choice that forces you to leave behind the multicolour world of grease and cheese to step into a green-coloured one filled with peculiar sounding vegetables like kale and healthy smoothies. You'd be surprised to know that the World Health Organization (WHO) has defined nutrition as 'the intake of food, following the body's dietary needs.'

Nutrition doesn't have to mean fancy, fitness-freaky food; all it means is a diet that consists of fresh and natural ingredients that fulfil your body's dietary needs. A fresh salad with colourful vegetables, home-made lentils and rice and a grilled chicken sandwich (sans the mayonnaise) are all examples of nutritious meals. A packaged granola health bar may contain high levels of sugar and saturated fats while home-cooked theplas and vegetables thrown on the grill can be an excellent way to get some lean protein and anti-inflammatory spices like cumin, fenugreek, and turmeric into your body. Simply put, WHO's philosophy that 'good nutrition—an adequate, well-balanced diet combined with regular physical activity—is a cornerstone of good health' is a good credo to not lose sight of.

Consider the meals you eat. What is the major part of your main meals: breakfast, lunch, and dinner? Do you realize that most of the time your meal is mostly wheat chapatti/ bread or white rice, which is accompanied by whatever else is on the menu, sometimes it is dal or a vegetable, an added curd or chutney/achaar.

Most of the time we just eat as a matter of habit. Have we thought that the chapatti we eat is primarily carbohydrates and every portion of carbohydrates that we eat should have an appropriate portion of protein (dairy and pulses), fat (ghee and oils) and vitamins and minerals (dairy, vegetables, salads, and chutneys)? Unless all these nutrients are eaten in a definite proportion, you are not eating a balanced diet.

To understand this better, consider the ICMR guidelines. As per this, an Indian sedentary adult male needs this ratio:

Cereals and millets	30 gms
Pulses	30 gms
Milk and milk products	100 ml
Roots and Tubers	100 gms
Green vegetables	100 gms
Other vegetables	100 gms
Fruits	100 gms
Sugar	5 gms
Fat	2.5 gms

This guideline clearly shows that we need to eat equal amounts of cereals and pulses, lots of milk, fruits, and vegetables to meet our recommended daily requirement of proteins, vitamins, and minerals.

Picture this:

For every 1 roti/chapatti (approx. 30 gms of wheat), you should consume:
1 cup of dal
½ cup of milk as curd/paneer
½ cup of green vegetables (like spinach, methi, lauki, torai, tinda, pepper, karela, cucumber)
½ cup of other vegetables (like tomato, brinjal, beans, onions, garlic, lotus stem, cauliflower, cabbage, broccoli)

½ cup of roots and tubers (like potato, sweet potato, arbi, yam)
½ tsp of healthy oilseed oil/ghee

You need to know this:

The 'multigrain' term used in commercially packaged food means only that more than one grain is present—and the primary ingredient is usually refined wheat flour.

The Confusion Surrounding Nutrition

There is no doubt that maintaining good health has become somewhat of an essential issue in the recent past. With lifestyle-related diseases like diabetes and heart ailments affecting more and more people the profession of nutritionists and dieticians has boomed beyond imagination. While nutritionists have helped a significant part of the world's population get its life back on track, they have also complicated food for the significant other. We live in the Internet age, and that means everybody has access to a mine of conflicting information. While the innocent potato and the somewhat comforting food group of fat have earned a bad reputation, various people have taken to adopting multiple diets. Right from the Paleo diet and Dukan diet to the Atkins and Keto diet, all everybody seems to want to do is lose weight.

Unfortunately, we have gotten all tangled up in this sticky web of speciality diets and 'healthy' ingredients that promise to burn our pockets. The focus has shifted from eating healthy to losing weight, and that translates to 'the end justifies all means' philosophy. Teenagers and young adults choose to cut carbohydrates, dairy, and all kind of fat from their diet in the desperate attempt to lose weight, forgetting that in these formative years of their lives, they are eliminating essential micronutrients required for bone formation and brain health.

As I consult individuals in the clinics or talk to multiple people at various platforms—conferences, sessions, and workshops—I am amazed at the fact that the questions still stay basic and simple. Many highly educated, well-read, and informed clients ask questions that show there is an overload of confusing and contradictory information.

- What oil should I use? Is ghee okay or is olive oil a better choice?
- Should I eat any fat in my diet or should I go on a fat-free diet?
- Is green tea better than my brewed masala tea (my masala tea makes me happy whereas green tea makes me grumpy)?
- Is it safe to use a sweetener, how many servings and which category of sweetener is the best?
- Should I drink cold-pressed vegetable juice or 100% Tetra Pak fruit juice?
- If I don't eat carbs at night, how do I sleep peacefully on a hungry, deprived stomach?

- Why is everybody shifting to chia seeds, are they better than the melon seeds I have?

This book attempts to answer such basic questions and links them to facts and our traditional cultural intelligence.

Few questions to ponder:
1. My grandmom had never heard of protein or the daily requirements, forget counting her protein intake on a daily basis. This notwithstanding she lived a healthy life, had healthy skin and hair and no major diseases.
2. Our parents did not buy avocados and blueberries but they instinctively knew that local seasonal fruits and vegetables had the power to keep all metabolic diseases at bay.
3. Our children for hundreds of years have grown up on a glass of milk—they could digest.

Somebody's Ignorance is Somebody's Gain

You need to know this:

Most fast-food is very high in sodium—even items you might think are not. For example, the veggie burger has 900 milligrams, followed by the corn muffin—770 milligrams. The shake has nearly twice as much sodium as the fries (530 vs. 290).

Fast-Foods

Fast-food may sound like a modern thing but its roots date back to early 1900s, thanks to a number of factors including modernization, mechanizations, feminist movements, increase in quality of life, social progress, and most importantly the World Wars. However, the market actually took off in the second half of the twentieth century when women shouldered the responsibility of a bread earner for the family. Entrepreneurs were quick to acknowledge that they had a consumer base in hand that had bucks to shell out but had scarcity of time to take care of their nutrition.

A study, titled *Food processing: a century of change*, published in the *Oxford Journals* stated:

"With the increasing standard of living, women soon understood that restaurants could be a good alternative to their home cooking. The feminist movements of the period proposed automated food chains and centralized kitchens, the main goal was to liberate women from the preparation of food that was time-consuming and, at the same time, very costly. The concept of ready-cooked food soon spread around the country. Fast-food describes food products that can be prepared and served very quickly."

Fast-food may be defined as any food which is ready-to-eat, whether a hot meal, burger, and chips, or ready-made chicken salad sandwich and a doughnut. Fast-food is more varied and of a higher quality than it was twenty years ago.

Nevertheless, a typical fast-food meal of cheeseburger and chips with apple pie and a large cola contains 1100 to 1200 calories. This amounts to 60% of the recommended daily calorie intake for the average seven- to ten-year-olds, with many of these calories coming out of the saturated fats and sugar. The cola alone, apart from its caffeine and colouring, contains more than eight teaspoons of sugar. Although such a meal is rich in macro or energy-dense nutrients, it tends to be low in essential micronutrients.

A diet based on fast-food is not a recipe for good health. It will probably not supply enough vitamin A, C, E, or sufficient amounts of trace minerals and fibre. The other problem with fast-food is that it 'crowds out' fresh fruits and vegetables. It tends to be high in fat (mainly saturated fat), sodium, or sugar and low in fibre. Consequently, eating fast-food in the diet increases obesity and related disorders such as heart disease and cancer.

The fast-food industry is increasing. McDonald's, the world's largest hamburger chain, serves at least 13000 customers a minute, or more than 98 million every week. This is not surprising since fast-food is so affordable and convenient for all ages. A survey has found that around 25% adolescents in India visit fast-food outlets once a week. But many dishes that one eats outside can be replicated at home, with a healthier twist. And that makes a lot of difference.

You need to know this:

- Tomato, cottage cheese (a firm white Indian cheese also known as paneer made from buffalo or cow milk) and avocado salad with warm homemade bread makes for a healthy meal.
- An omelette with fresh herbs takes three minutes to prepare and two minutes to cook. Served with green salad or fresh vegetables and a wholemeal roll, it provides a perfectly balanced meal.
- Beans, vegetable and ginger stir-fry with rice noodles take just ten minutes to prepare and provide a right balance of vital nutrients.

By choosing foods carefully from fast-food menus, you can select a reasonably well-balanced meal, while limiting the intake of more harmful ingredients. For instance, choose small plain burgers as opposed to a giant burger with all the trimmings. Or skip the mayonnaise and melted cheese. By leaving these out, 200 calories can be saved on a king-sized burger (also reduces your fat intake). Or order milk instead of a milkshake, or just plain water instead of a conventional cola drink. If you are having fries, choose a smaller portion and have a side salad. And never be persuaded to eat massive helpings than you need.

And the Aftermath

People often believe that if the life expectancy of our population is higher and we're living longer, then we're mostly healthier. However, this statistical deduction is a little misleading.

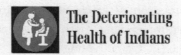

The Deteriorating Health of Indians

There are 69.1 million people with diabetes in India, according to the International Diabetes Federation— India is now the diabetes capital of the world.

India is home to 9.8 million obese men and 20 million fat women, according to a study published in The Lancet journal in 2014. Obesity is on the rise, especially in metro cities like Mumbai, Delhi, and Bangalore.

An average Indian consumes 10.98 grams of salt per day— 119% more than the recommended limit of five grams per day by the World Health Organization.

26% of all deaths in India happen due to cardiovascular diseases.

The common factors tying non-communicable lifestyle diseases are unhealthy eating patterns and a lack of physical exercise. People today are ageing at a never-seen-before rate. Premature greying and balding are especially prevalent in men; hypertension and diabetes are striking people in their twenties. While it is true that hypertension runs in families, doctors maintain that it can also be solely related to unhealthy habits such as excessive smoking, drinking, and a sedentary lifestyle. High-stress levels and long working hours is another factor that makes younger people susceptible to obesity and diabetes. Experts have repeatedly stressed the mounting patterns of stress among youth and teenagers. Unprecedented levels of stress are the primary cause of premature greying, dark circles, and Polycystic Ovary Syndrome (PCOS) in young adults.

The humble dabba—tiffin—has been replaced by my more attractive options like canteen pav bhaji and vada pav or some quick Chinese food laden with Ajinomoto from the stall across the street. Leisurely walks have been replaced with Netflix marathons, and Internet browsing and your mother's fruit cream and halwa have been replaced with treats such as waffles, pancakes, and freakshakes, all rich in high levels of sugar and refined flour. It is terrible foods like these which are high in unhealthy LDL cholesterol that causes adults to get caught up in a tangle of lifestyle disorders, some that are often irreversible.

Hypertension, obesity, and diabetes together spell high risk for severe cardiovascular diseases. The good news? Healthy eating and regular exercise have found to improve such conditions and even protect patients with hypertension from becoming susceptible to cardiac arrests. Metabolic disorders, especially diabetes 1 and 2, are another area of concern that's affecting the populations like wildfire.

Profit Over Health: The Pharma Industry

International crime, faulty and often fraud testing of drugs, and negligence in ensuring safe manufacturing of drugs—the pharma industry is one of the biggest law-breaking rackets in the world. Pharmaceutical industries—which today generate revenue at the same pace as Wall Street—go to great lengths to mislead health authorities about the safety of their products. An upcoming trend is the 'recycling of drugs' by bigger pharma companies—hiking prices only to pump repurposed drugs back into the market.

History suggests that as the pharmaceutical industry grew bigger and reached its peak, alliances formed between pharma companies and physicians. This meant that essential and noted medical practices were quick to dispose of doctors who chose a non-pharmacologically based medicine that was now considered ineffective and non-profitable.

The fact remains that medication only takes you halfway to the finishing line. It is a healthy diet and proper nutrition that get you through all the way. Just before the advent of the pharma industry in the first half of the twentieth century, doctors realized that food contained specific properties that could fight sickness. Orphans and prisoners who suffered from aggressive rashes and dementia aka pellagra could be helped by including niacin in their diets; increasing deaths of sailors after long oceanic voyages due to a mysterious disease aka scurvy could be prevented by eating citrus fruits and vegetables—proof of the magical healing powers of food.

Most people believe that anxiety and stress can best be dealt with medication and drugs. However, one of the most influential weapons to combat anxiety comes not from the chemist but the grocer. Foods rich in zinc such as oysters, peanuts, sesame, horse gram, pumpkin seeds, cashews, liver, beef, and egg yolks have been linked to lowered anxiety. Other foods, including fatty fish like wild Alaskan salmon, contain omega-3 fatty acid. A study completed on medical students in 2011 was one of the first to show that omega-3 may help reduce anxiety. Believe it or not, you can eat your way to a better state of mind.

Pharmaceutical companies research, develop, and exploit drugs to prevent, control, and cure diseases and treat symptoms. Companies then market these medications to recover their investments and reward shareholders. It would seem to serve the interests of society, but it is a vicious circle in which businesses invent new diseases to match their existing drugs. Increasingly, the industry has found itself under fire from detractors who contend that, in the pursuit of profits, companies are in league with medical doctors and patient advocacy groups to convince people that their usually mild ailment urgently needs drug treatment.

Have you wondered about a worrying trend: Pharma companies have drugs for every ailment? Sales of these companies are skyrocketing. Healthcare is becoming more and more organized. Large cities in India have hundreds of hospitals. But is all this resulting in better health or are we seeing more sickness? The fact is that many illnesses are preventable with good diet and lifestyle and before a person pops a pill to manage a symptom or disease, he should reflect more on his food, lifestyle, and schedules.

The Nutrition Gap: Medication Is Not The Solution

The pharmaceutical industry may be king, but nutrition trumps all. All over the world, the traditional medical approach has been to focus on treatment than on the prevention of diseases. In fact, for the better part of the last century, the standard medical curriculum only spends a few days in the four years of training on discussing how nutrition and wellness affect the progression of the disease. Most of the education focuses on medication, testing, and surgery. While procedure mainly entails medical help, prevention has more to do with a diet fortified by whole grains and fresh vegetables. Think of your body as a washbasin, until the drain has been cleared it isn't fit for usage. Simply put, until your body flushes out illness-causing toxins, there is little purpose in pumping it with medication.

Doctors have been trained and incentivized to work for sick-care rather than health-care, and although a proper diet is known to bring heart-wellness, doctors focus more on the drugs rather than discussing the nutrition change that the patient can make. A simple example of this attitude is an average doctor's prescribed treatment for a patient with calcium deficiency. Often, when a patient complains of bone ache and fatigue, the doctor suspecting osteoporosis, recommends a DXA scan (alias DXA scans are used to measure bone density and assess the risk of bone fractures) and writes down a list of calcium supplements to be taken. At no point during the appointment is the patient told why the scan is required and why exactly are calcium levels low. A conversation regarding the patient's dietary plan and ways to increase calcium through food seldom takes place; the quick-fix is always medication.

Nearly half of the adults in the world take at least one prescription medicine, as diseases such as obesity, diabetes, and heart ailments grow more prevalent. The problem with medicating illnesses such as hypertension and elevated cholesterol is that the drugs treat symptoms without addressing the cause—diet. Overmedicated, and even malnourished, most of us fail to understand that the answer to the treatment of diseases doesn't lie in more tablets but in the food that we consume daily. With so much incorrect and conflicting nutritional information regarded as 'general knowledge', from 'all-protein' to 'no egg yolks', the average person is unaware of the deadly effects of packaged convenience foods that are not only devoid of nutrition but also invite disease.

The simple fact is that medication is a short-term solution that only alleviates symptoms, an instant formula to solve all problems. Only insulin injections will not treat diabetes; a healthy and low-sugar diet is the key to a speedy recovery. A protein-rich diet and regular physical exercise have shown to cause a significant improvement in patients who have diabetes. Monitoring salt intake and consuming water-rich foods has proven to be beneficial for people with hypertension. A nutritious diet is a way to live a hale and hearty life, and it is time that doctors have a conversation that can save your life. In the same way that cars are designed to operate on specific kinds of fuel, so is the human body intended to work on particular types of healthy foods.

You need to know this:

One of the first drugs to come into common usage, aspirin, is still one of the most researched medicines in the world, with an estimated 700 to 1,000 clinical trials conducted each year.

Damage Control: Key Message And The Way Forward

Fortunately for us Indians, our daily diet gives us all the nourishment we need. Our lunch, composed of whole-wheat chapattis, legumes, and freshly-cooked, spiced vegetables is a one-meal wonder. In a nutshell, all I can say that our ancestors were right and traditional foods are the way to go.

So what counts as traditional food? Food that nourished the evolution of our ancestors before industrialization came along in the nineteenth century and transformed diet to the atrocity that we know it as today. In the simplest terms, traditional food is based on four principles:

1) Abstinence from refined foods.
2) A celebration of whole and natural grains.
3) Recognizing the importance of nutrition in our lives.
4) Preparing meals in the same way that nourished our. ancestors. Eat only that food that your grandmother would approve of.

Diseases like infertility, diabetes, and obesity were mostly non-existent in cultures surviving on a native diet of unrefined foods. Unfortunately, in this age of readily available convenience foods like frozen cheesy snacks, frozen cuts of meat, and ready-to-eat meals, we tend to get busy with our careers and forget to take care of ourselves. Fact is that convenience foods aren't all that convenient for your health. Regular snacking on foods high in sodium, excess salt, and sugar has replaced family meals eaten fresh on the dining table. The dabba system that not only helped you make friends with the surly boss whose only weakness was aate ka halwa also helped you keep your heart healthy. Today that dabba has been replaced with three-minute ready-to-eat meals that sit on the shelves of supermarket stores, beaming with pride for their immortality. We have moved to the grab-and-go age of food, food containing high amounts of hidden sugar, sodium, and preservatives that almost always translate into dangerous consequences for the future.

Now is the time to take control of your lives, go ahead and have the nutrition conversation that can change your life. Clear your cupboards of instant noodles, sugar-laden biscuits, and the greasy packet of Haldiram aloo bhujia; a new era of healthy, whole grain snacks is here to save the day. After all, whole food leads to entire health.

Try any of the meals given below when the munchies strike:

- Switch the maida/refined flour for ragi or jowar flour the next time you make Sunday pancakes. The high amount of dietary fibre in ragi has shown to lower blood sugar levels and helps in weight loss.
- Craving the greasy golden goodness of McDonald's French fries? Make sweet potato oven-baked fries at home instead. Giving you the same crunch and satisfaction, this snack will provide you with twice the amount of fibre than regular white potatoes and is super rich in potassium.
- The sweltering heat and sweet cravings giving you no rest? Refrigerate two bananas overnight and chuck them in a blender the next morning with some honey and blueberries. Voila, you get creamy, smooth ice cream that is rich in anti-oxidants and potassium.
- Cannot resist the buttery call of salty, crunchy movie hall popcorn? No worries, get yourself a packet of fresh corn seeds from an organic store, pop in a vessel with butter and some garlic for a tastier, healthier alternative.

In this book, I invite the reader to have a conversation about what defines good health and proper nutrition and debunk myths about so-called 'bad' foods born out of the menace of medical misinformation. In this book, you will find information on growingly prevalent diseases like diabetes, hypertension, and heart diseases that seem to have confounded doctors.

Nutrition seems to have lost its place in the world today. The aim of this book is to give a healthy and nutritious diet the recognition it deserves. Backed by my experience, the book details the impact dietary choices have on our health and how medication is not always the right answer. Accompanied by suggestions, recipes, and advice, the book guides the reader to find the path that leads to a healthy life—one that is most certainly built using the bricks of nutrition.

Before you flip to the next chapter, let's do some goal setting:

Goals	I will	I won't	Maybe
Eat right			
Lose extra body fat			
Read about food			
Change food habits			
Sleep properly			
Medical check-ups on time			
Wash and eat fruits and vegetables			

Goals	I will	I won't	Maybe
Eat cooked and raw food			
Avoid sugar and white flour			
Avoid processed, packaged food			
Have one healthy morning ritual			

CHAPTER TWO

Your Friends' Perspective: Lose Those Extra Pounds, My Friend!

Mondays are usually sunny and high on energy. Not for everyone, though! Not everyone is keen on going for a session at the gym on a Monday morning. Most of us even skip breakfast because our alarms do not buzz at the right time. And not eating lunch to keep up with work schedules is just a small compromise. All the people in their late twenties and early thirties who are tied to corporate nuances and instruments like laptops and handhelds have no time for a morning meal. Their idea is to have a cup of tea with maybe a toast and almost no butter. Butter makes you fat! That's the thought that goes around.

Below are two case studies. The first one is a perfect example of how our elaborate strategies and plans on weight loss begin with coffee-table discussions and dies at 'Oh God! I am so busy to follow this'. While the second one underscores the plight of a helpless to-be-married man whose would-be wife wants him to lose weight. Before we start discussing the relevance of these two studies, let's first see what they are up to.

Case I

Rashmi, a thirty-two-year-old, has a theory. A dashing investment banker, Rashmi is good with numbers and better with her eating habits. She has always been conscious of what she eats and her exercise routine—she may compromise on her sleep but never on her workout session. An inspiration to everyone who knows her, she has been pushing her friends—Niharika, Komal, and Drishti—to take up a proper work-out regime and eat healthy.

Komal, a typical Indian housewife, cannot control the oil in her food. Her usual excuse is: 'How can I use less oil while cooking a meal? How will a vegetable be cooked in just that much?' And Drishti, a social media manager, cannot control her diet of chocolates. Chocolates are her first love and even a Lindt, which says 75% dark chocolate, is a daily snack for her. She'd rather carry more Lindt than MAC in her bag, because 'you need more chocolates than make-up'. Niharika does not know what to choose and what to eat. Her diet is a mixture of some fantastic snacks, and wheat flour is the first choice! But having the work schedule of a banker, her eating habits are irregular and her caffeine intake alarmingly high.

Today, they have taken out a day from their busy schedules to meet up with Rashmi and discuss their weight loss issues.

Rashmi waits for them at Starbucks, sipping her decaf, low-fat cappuccino with brown sugar, comfortably avoiding the chocolate cookies served along with it. She flips through her social media and taps open a health video from a fitness brand on Facebook. The video offers a recent insight into the wheat intake. A minute into the video, Komal calls her, shouting on the phone: "Hey Rashmi! Can't find you! Where are you?"

"I am sitting on the corner left table at Starbucks."

"Oh! Is Starbucks it? All right! Give us five minutes."

The call disconnects and Rashmi continues to watch the video. She finishes her coffee. The cookies, however, lie in loneliness on the table thinking about their friend, coffee, who has already been on the trail and has vanished from the cup without them. They feel dejected for there seem to be no takers for them. The cookies are sad!

Komal has just entered the café followed by Niharika and Drishti.

Niharika, as expected, is enamoured by the sandwiches and cakes on the shelf. They seem like Diwali lights to her. They lure her with their colours and flavours. She gazes at the menu and back to the shelf where a plethora of food is lying to be claimed. She cannot stop herself from ordering a banana cake and has lost her friends in the crowded Starbucks.

Once she has ordered, she somehow manages to find Rashmi.

"Hey! Wait, where are Komal and Drishti?" asks Rashmi, getting up to greet her.

As Rashmi and Niharika hug and sit down, Niharika is quick in claiming the abandoned cookies. The cookies have finally found their love. Komal, who had taken a detour to the washroom, rushes in to hug Rashmi and announces to Drishti, who follows behind her, and Niharika: 'See, I told you she wouldn't eat the cookies. I know this girl. Too much of a health fanatic.'

Drishti is seeing Rashmi after a while, and is amazed by her appearance. "Look at you, Rash! How did you lose those love handles? What are you now, a size 6 or what?"

As the four sit down, Komal begins, "This Bombay traffic, I tell you. Such a waste of time. We could have met at my place. That would have been easier. But it's okay. I can pick up Nirvana from school. Anyway, how are you, Rashmi? See! That weight loss remedy isn't helping at all. I have done it for a good three weeks now. I do not see any change in my figure. The weight monitor still clocks 71 kgs. I do not think it is working for me. I have a different body type than yours."

"Banana cake and java chip frappuccino for Niharika!" shouts the waiter. Niharika jumps up and rushes to the counter to take her order.

Komal and Rashmi gaze at Drishti.

Rashmi: "When did she place that order?"

Drishti: "I have no freaking idea!"

Komal: "Leave it. Tell me how do I become fit in the next one month? I have to attend my sister's wedding and I am freaking out! That dress won't accommodate my curves. Rashmi, please help me!"

"You don't eat right. How do I help you with that?" asks Rashmi.

Komal gasps and after a long moment, says, "I have been trying my best. I cannot eat breakfast because there is always so much work at home. Manoj has to go to work at eight, then Nikita's school is at ten and—"

Rashmi interrupts her. "I am sure you can wake up a little early."

Meanwhile, Niharika is gazing at her mouth-watering banana cake and scouting for a private corner to take the first bite, so it gives her that feeling of contentment which food always gives her.

Drishti jokes at Komal's expense. "This lady cannot get up early. Her morning kick starts at eight when Manoj starts shouting about his tie and shoes!"

Komal: "That is not true, Drishti! Guys, I am trying. It is just that I cannot go on early morning walks and follow an exercise regime. Do not have the time. The household chores do not let me plan for a workout. What else can I do?"

Niharika, who is back on the table, gulps her java chip frappuccino and says, "Eat this"—pointing towards the banana cake—"and everything will be fine."

Komal rubbishes her and holds Rashmi's hand. "You got to help me in this weight loss. There is no time left for the wedding."

Niharika interrupts, saying, "Nothing works, guys. Komal, you have followed that yoga program for about a month. Even ordered that special foam mattress from US Amazon. Where is the bed now?"

"Nothing works for me!" Komal exhales helplessly.

Rashmi, who has been patiently hearing her friends up till now, cuts in: "Niharika, you keep enjoying your banana loads-of-calorie cake. You never really follow any routine, so you cannot complain about becoming obese! And Komal, you need to follow a strict diet, else the wedding and weight loss will be a dream!"

Drishti chimes in with an idea: "Why don't we all join some swimming classes together? Maybe in the evening after our husbands are back home?"

Niharika gulps another sip of her drink and says, "Sounds boring but count me in."

"Can't!" says Komal.

"Why not now?" questions Drishti.

Rashmi promptly replies, "Madam, she cannot miss her daily soaps. That is why!"

Komal interrupts, "No, it is not that. Just that it won't be possible after Manoj is home . . . What if I shift to a ketone diet? My neighbour's daughter has been following it and I saw her this morning and, my God, she has become a size 6 from a size 8!"

Rashmi: "Look at you, Komal. You cannot blindly follow a keto or a GM diet and lose weight. Do you even know what exactly a ketogenic diet regimen is?"

Komal is clueless, and so are Niharika and Drishti.

Looking at their faces, Rashmi continues, "A naturally ketogenic diet is a low-carb diet, but it's not just that. The regimen enables your body to primarily burn fat instead of carbohydrates. And mind you, it's a high-fat protein-rich diet so you might gain a couple of kilos in the beginning which is where people start to panic and leave the regimen, and then they nag about it. This is why one needs to make a strategy for a light work-out as well when on a ketogenic diet. Have patience and be strict in following it. One significant aspect of the food is fasting for 12-14 hours. Can you think of doing that, Komal?"

Komal reacts as if she is caught sleeping in the classroom. "What?" I mean, ummm . . ."

"See that's why it's essential for you to consider every aspect of the regimen you're going to follow," continues Rashmi. "I'm not saying that you should not do it, but the question is can you strictly follow it? Otherwise, you will just keep complaining about how this regimen didn't work for you."

Komal looks worried.

"To manage your routine better you can either take up binge eating or segment your eating hours according to your family routine. Take up fasting and eat fibre and fruits and drink ample water. Setting a food intake routine will help you get fit quickly. Does that make sense?" asks Rashmi. This time Komal nods in amazement and so do Niharika and Drishti.

Rashmi continues addressing everybody. "This fasting is necessary as it catalyses the body to make ketones from fat and utilizes them as fuel for energy. The process is also known as ketosis. The entire collection switches its fuel supply to fat. And as the fat metabolism increases dramatically, the excess fat stored in the body burns off efficiently thereby reducing the weight. And guess what? This isn't the end of this story, there are other less obvious benefits as well, such as less hunger and a steady supply of energy."

"What will I cook, Rashmi?" asks Komal slightly confused.

"You can find hundreds of recipes from dietdoctor. com," tells Rashmi.

"How about I ban sugar in my diet and eat no rice and just have one meal a day?" asks Komal, a little subdued.

Drishti and Rashmi let out a short giggle, as Komal sounds terribly cute to them.

Niharika jokes, "You will need some medical treatment by the end of the week!"

Rashmi affirms. "She is actually right! You can't just think of some random plan and lose weight. It is a continuous process, and everything counts. Further, studies have shown that you reduce 2.2 times more weight on a ketogenic diet than being on a calorie-restricted diet. Another study found out that people on the ketogenic diet lost three times more weight than those following Diabetes Recommended Diet."

Drishti pitches her point too. "But exercise helps a lot."

Rashmi clarifies promptly. "It does. Statistically speaking, jumping ropes, doing lunges, squats, high knees, and holding plank are few of the home exercises that burn calories the most. But you need to have a good diet regimen and follow a certain plan. Both go hand in hand. You cannot just walk 10 miles every day or do 100 squats but eat samosa and chutney and think you will lose weight. You also need to eat right!"

"And drink!" yells Niharika.

Komal yells back. "You better keep your theory to yourself. By the way, how is the cake? Less sugar?" And leans in to take a bite.

Rashmi and Drishti look at each other and pass a smile at Komal.

Still eating, Komal murmurs, "How about a surgery?"

Rashmi stops her then and there. "Do not even think about that. You don't need one."

Komal sadly points out, "I guess nothing's going to work. This is my body type and I should accept it. I will probably get a new dress. This does not work. Probably after Nikita, I couldn't lose further. This is what an abdominal surgery does to your body. No?"

Rashmi and Drishti nod in affirmation as Niharika takes the last sip of her coffee.

All four are still puzzled by the theory and execution of weight loss. For Rashmi, the inspiration in the group, it isn't clear as to how she should help Komal lose weight for the wedding while Niharika does not care and thinks it is what it is. Drishti's vague ideas find no takers.

The overall consensus is that nothing works, and one may do whatever he/she feels like but in the end one must accept one's body type, and if he/she has undergone an abdominal surgery then this weight concern is for life! Such instances and memories form a judgment, and people give up their routines.

The fact is that there are a lot of diet regimens available with dieticians and a lot freely available on the internet as well, such as ketogenic diet, GMT diet, and Paleo diet; however, one needs to be stringent in following it. All of these diet plans work provided one is willing to curb their craving for fried, processed, or carbohydrate-rich food.

One thing that overweight and obese people need to understand is that there are no shortcuts to weight reduction. There is no diet regimen that can single-handedly help you reduce 5-7 kgs in a week or 15 kgs in a month. Cardiac exercises like running on the treadmill or walking are also necessary for quick results.

Statistics show that 47% of people quit weight loss programs after the first week itself and the other 43% by the end of three weeks. Only 5% of people maintain a long-term weight loss regimen. Few of the primary reasons are hectic work schedule, no accountability, expensive training, too many expectations too soon, and, the most significant reason, lack of motivation, secondary only to boring and monotonous workouts.

Every problem has a solution. Start slowly. Before you even go on a strict regimen, start avoiding junk food and snacking. Meanwhile, start substituting cooked vegetables with unprocessed meat and salad and gradually come on a stringent diet. Give yourself at least two weeks before you start seeing the results. Talking about lack of motivation, how about the fact that obesity is the primary reason for type 2 diabetes, pulmonary oedema, hypertension, fatigue, back pain neuropathy and what not?

'Health is wealth,' and it all starts with eating well and maintaining a healthy BMI. Lack of self-monitoring is the most significant reason why people become obese in the first place. Craving and binge eating is the most prominent cause of obesity, and this can be easily avoided. One needs to get rid of all the distractions while eating, start intuitive eating, and always be well hydrated. One point which is not emphasized enough is that one ought to drink water 15-20 minutes before a meal and 40 minutes after having lunch, ensuring that the fat and protein are metabolized more efficiently.

It's the time to put on your dancing shoes, or as you might call them your workout boots, and hit the road. Play some music while you walk or exercise to enjoy the time. Garnish your food with some black pepper or healthy toppings to add some taste to your healthy eating. Make a strategy!

Case II

Udbhav and Saarika are happily married. Both fell in love during their college years and later, after the consent and blessings of their elders, got married. They are now planning for their first child. Saarika works in a reputed public sector bank while her husband successfully runs his business venture. There is a lot happening in Saarika's life at the moment as her friend, Advika, is about to get married to Subodh.

Saarika has been especially as well as specifically asked to look after all the arrangements related to her friend's wedding, to which she has readily agreed. Since both the ladies are incredibly conscious about their health and physique, with Advika being a health fanatic, there is entirely no compromise on the health front.

But Subodh has gone a little plump around the belly lately, something Advika doesn't appreciate at all. In a bid to make her fiancé lost weight, she even mock threatened to get the marriage postponed. If and whenever asked, Subodh says that it's because of Advika's family members, especially her mother and sisters, who force-feed him nearly all kinds of food items that Advika doesn't even touch. And the reason behind it is the obvious one: "You are not eating enough . . . You appear thin and weak!" Typical treatment of a son-in-law at her wife's or wife-to-be's home!

Therefore, Subodh has decided to have a casual chat with Saarika and her husband so that either they can talk Advika out of her current mock threat (he isn't too sure!) or help him become what she wants him to. Although Subodh is also a health-conscious guy but the love he has been showered with recently combined with a rigorous schedule during the work hours has given an unpleasant transformation to his body; one even he abhors completely.

A weekend is chosen and Sunday fixed for the chat between Saarika, Udbhav, and Subodh.

Excited for the talks, Subodh reaches a full hour early. The couple is happily surprised to receive him early, and when told, Subodh says, "It's good then, na? More time for talks!"

They both give in to his excitement. Saarika comes out with cups of green tea, seeing which Subodh gives an expression that shows how unenthusiastic he is to the idea of green tea. Saarika is quick to realize it and asks, "Regular tea or coffee for you, then?"

Subodh nearly chuckles at the offer and says, "Yes, please!"

But to his surprise Udbhav interrupts. "Therein lies the problem. You already know it's not good for health because of the caffeine content, but still, you laid down your arms. You must not surrender to such cravings of yours so soon and that too so easily."

Saarika adds: "Udbhav's correct. Have green tea; it will help you burn a few extra calories."

Having no other possible choice, Subodh picks up the cup and takes a big sip. "It's quite good, thanks!"

Saarika continues; "So, have I heard correctly that Advika has threatened to postpone the date of the wedding?"

Subodh blushes a bit and says, "Yes, she did say something like this, but I'm not considering it as a serious threat. Wait. She won't do that, right?"

Saarika laughs. "As far as I know Advika, she can, mister. You better not treat that as a hollow threat."

"Stop making him feel even more miserable, just help him out and work your magic as you did on me," Udbhav chimes in.

Saarika nods and asks Subodh, "What's your day-to-day routine like?"

Subodh: "Well, I usually get up around seven in the morning and then after freshening up I take up some light exercising for about half an hour. After that I have a bath, then breakfast, before finally leaving for office. Due to a lot of office work, I mostly skip my lunchtime meal. I return around 6 in the evening and prefer going for a walk for about 15-20 minutes. Then I have dinner around 9. After that, I sit down to finish my official work. Finally, I sleep around 11 or so."

Udbhav: "Wow! You summarized that very well."

Saarika: "This is about what you do. What I'm interested in is what you have."

Subodh: "For breakfast, it's mostly potato-stuffed sandwiches though sometimes I also have oats. As I told you earlier, I skip lunch most of the times. Dinner is light and usually roti, rice, and dal."

Saarika: "What then for beverages and how many times a day?"

Subodh, already feeling somewhat guilty: "Normal caffeine tea 2-3 times at home and about 3-4 mugs of coffee at the office . . . per day"

Udbhav: "That's quite a lot . . . It has visibly taken a toll on your health."

Saarika: "Listen, Subodh, let me suggest a few things. You exercise in the morning, and that's appreciable, but you still have to give up a lot of negative health practices and adopt a few healthier ones."

Subodh: "Hmm."

Saarika: "Try to wake up a bit earlier in the morning, anytime around or before 6 would do. Have lukewarm water with honey and some kick of lemon. Shift your schedule of evening walks and make them morning ones instead."

Subodh: "Why so?"

Udbhav: "Morning fresh air is good for a healthy metabolism and lungs while the air around evening hours is usually heavily polluted. So, instead of doing any good, it worsens your health. Also, the time you are spending on evening walks, you can try swimming for that duration. It will burn a lot of extra calories and fat from your body!"

Subodh: "That's an excellent scientific update and alternative, thanks. What else?"

Saarika: "Do NOT skip lunch! Make it a rule of life never to skip breakfast and lunch. Your indulgence in exhaustive works without proper meals will surely harm you."

Subodh: "All right, I'll have lunch starting tomorrow. Even if it's a small meal, I'll surely try to have something rather work on an empty stomach. Then?"

Saarika: "Include sprouts in your breakfast along with some seasonal fruits, juices, and dry fruits like walnut. Oats are good. Start a ketogenic diet which is a low-carb diet. But it's not just that, the regimen enables your body to primarily burn fat instead of carbohydrates. But, it's a high-fat protein-rich diet, so you might gain some weight in the beginning."

Subodh: "What? Gain? I came all the way here to seek the advice on losing some kilos, and you are telling me to adopt a diet that will add some!"

Udbhav: "The gain is only an initial phase, as your body begins to burn fat, you'll witness the difference yourself. Moreover, with saved carbohydrates, you won't need the coffee breaks anymore. You'll have ample energy to work without the intake of caffeine."

Subodh: "I should better write all this down somewhere. Forgetting even a point of what both of you are advising might postpone my marriage!"

Saarika (to Udbhav, laughing): "His eagerness to get married reminds me of you! Here, have this pen and paper.

"And Subodh, it's essential for you to reconsider every aspect of the regimen you're going to follow. I'm not saying that you shouldn't follow it, but the question is can you strictly practice it? Otherwise, you will keep complaining about how this regimen didn't work for you."

Subodh: "Anything for Advika!"

Saarika: "Aww . . . What love! Advika is a lucky girl. Moreover, you can try segmentation of your diet hours."

Subodh: "Anything else, ma'am?"

Saarika: "With a ketogenic diet, a bit of fasting is also required. This fasting is necessary as it catalyses the body to make ketones from fat and uses them as fuel for energy. The entire body switches its fuel supply to stored fat. And as the fat metabolism increases, the excess stored in the body burns off thereby reducing the weight. Can you do it?"

Subodh: "Well, I was skipping lunch until now. I can switch to light dinner instead, will that count as fasting?"

Saarika and Subodh: "In a subtle way, yes. But don't ease up on the physical workout. Otherwise, you'll be back to square one."

Subodh: "I'll keep that I mind. Thanks a lot, guys. You've been a huge help to me."

Udbhav: "You're always welcome, my friend."

Subodh: "And what do I owe you for such a wonderful session, ma'am? I mean your consultation charges?"

Saarika (laughing): "Keep my sister-like friend happy . . . I demand nothing else."

Subodh: "I've already made that promise to Advika. I'll live by it. Thanks, I'll take your leave now."

Saarika: "All right, take care. Don't hesitate to contact us if you require any help regarding anything."

Subodh: "I will. Why spend my money elsewhere when I have both of you!"

As we saw, different people have different weight loss woes. While somebody wants to fit into her wedding gown, somebody may want to look dashing on his wedding. But the reason that everybody should be interested in to stay healthy. Because weight gain is just the beginning of health problems and it's better to start before it is too late.

The common problem in both of the above scripts was the gap between the planning and execution. There are many ways to lose weight including all the diets we discussed above including ketogenic diet, GMT diet, and Paleo diet. But, the question is who will bell the cat. All these diets require strict dietary discipline as well as a tight physical activity schedule, something which many could not even begin with. And those who begin, lose way in a couple of days.

The idea is no matter what way you choose to achieve weight loss, you should not lose it until you do it.

Findings from the latest *American Journal of Clinical Nutrition* study suggest six key strategies for long-term success at weight loss:

1) engaging in high levels of physical activity
2) eating a diet that is low in calories and fat

3) eating breakfast
4) self-monitoring weight on a regular basis
5) maintaining a consistent eating pattern
6) catching 'slips' before they turn into larger regains

Goal Setting:

My Weekly Planner
- **Let's see your progress in one month**

Goals	Week 1	Week 2	Week 3	Week 4	
Exercise and walk for 30-45 minutes					
3 meals and 2 small snacks					
Restrict coffee to 2 cups					
Eat 4 servings of fruits					
Sleep for at least 6 hours each day					
Switch off your phone an hour before bedtime					
At least 1 serving of whole beans/sprouts					
Dinner before 7:30					

Goals	Week 1	Week 2	Week 3	Week 4	
Stayed away from Cheese Cookies Bread					
Replaced unhealthy snacks with roasted nuts					

** Give yourself 1 mark for each goal that you are able to achieve.

- Score less than 5: Oh! You missed it.
- Score 5-7: You are up to something.
- Score 7 and above: Almost there!
- Perfect 10: Congrats! You're a health enthusiast.

Health Disclaimer: The above goal setting is only to help you get aligned to a healthy routine. On the basis of the above chart, you can make your own goals depending on your aspiration and limitations and follow it for a healthier life.

DOs, when you are on a diet	DON'Ts when you are on a diet
Eat at 3 fixed times with an interval of 5-6 hours	Avoid repeated snacking
Keep yourself well-hydrated	Avoid soda drinks

DOs, when you are on a diet	DON'Ts when you are on a diet
Very important to fast for 14 hours when on a ketogenic diet	Do not eat fruits like apples, bananas, oranges, and mangoes when on a ketogenic diet
Light cardiac exercise like treadmill or cycling will go a long way in helping you reduce weight	Never skip breakfast

Goal setting: And you thought weight loss was easy!?

Worry pointers	Your 12th Man!
How to reduce simple carbs?	Replace bread with wheat or pancakes. Eat poha/upma instead of muesli. Replace white sugar with brown.
How about our Physical Activity?	Take up a physical routine. Either walk a mile or perform some activity.
How much should you sleep?	Beauty sleep is 6-8 hours. Rest is your call.
Eat this! Not that!	Cut down on the juice, cheese, boxed eatables, and choose naturals like ghee, poha, besan pancake, buttermilk, nuts, bhuna chana, for a better diet.

Worry pointers	Your 12th Man!
Relax to not Re-lapse.	Throw stress out of the window to relax. Take up meditation and breathe easy.

Well, you should count these too!

Hot-shots	Calorie bites
Cookies (8 gms)	Two cookies mean 80 calories. Unfriend, right away!
2 pieces of bread and 1 tablespoon of butter	220 calories! Try looking away when it is served.
Namkeen (2 spoons)	Namkeens have a wide range. It is usually between 100 cal. (2 spoons) to 150 cal. Next time, sip your tea instead.
Caramel chocolate	Well, 1 square is 35 calories. I am sure you can do the math!
Cappuccino	100 calories and I am not even counting caffeine.
Subway	Your sub is hygienically prepared but calorie intake ranges from 100-150 in a 6-inch sub. Unfriend this one too!
Pickles	Hate to share this number but 15 grams of mango pickle is 40 calories. Fact!

Handy tips for a healthy eating regimen:

1. An egg isn't your 'cholesterol-enemy': Eggs have about 2 grams of saturated fat, which is only 10% of the daily value and no trans fat.
2. Avoid HFCS or High Fructose Corn Sugar: HFCS is worse than sugar. It is a mimic of sucrose in composition and action. Packed juices, flavoured yoghurt, bread, sauces contain HFCS. It is no better!
3. No raw food provides enzymes that are required for a healthy digestion: Food cooked above 47 degrees inactivates most enzymes and is not useful for our digestion. Plant enzymes are protein in nature. Eat raw and cooked food but cook mildly to protect plant enzymes.
4. Calories taken after sunset are more fattening than the ones taken during the day: Myth. Bust it. Any calorie is a bad calorie, but eat them in the evening only when there is an activity associated after the meal.
5. My weight problem is because my body does not process wheat or dairy that I eat.

Remember, half knowledge is dangerous. Think positively. Problems are plenty and so are the solutions. Always consult an expert and simply follow his or her advice.

So What Works?

- **Drink lots of water:** Do not confuse thirst with hunger.
- **Watch for portion size:** Eat several small meals during the day.
- **Do not skip meals:** Never skip breakfast.
- **Eat at least 5 servings of fruits and vegetables per day:** Packed with beneficial fibres, vitamins, and antioxidants, these also help keep your calorie count low.
- **Go for wholesome fresh foods:** Purchase fresh foods and avoid packaged, processed and convenient foods such as fast-food, tinned, canned, frozen, ready-to-eat food.
- **Understand Food Claims and Labels:** Product labelled with a fat-free claim does not mean that it is low in calories.
- **Protein at every meal:** Eating high-quality protein maintains muscle mass and reduces body fat during weight loss.
- **Take control of emotional eating:** In a state of stress, loneliness, or depression, try to not eat unhealthy or binge eat.
- **Keep a food journal (plan and follow your own menu):** This helps you pinpoint your eating pattern and will enable you to easily modify it.
- **Don't be overly-restrictive:** Simply allow yourself

a little indulgence, but watch out for the frequency and the quantity.

- **Exercise:** Try 30-60 minutes of physical activity a day to stay healthy. If you wish to lose weight, then you'll have to exercise more.
- **Buddy up:** Getting support from others to maintain your new eating and physical activity habits.
- **Choose your portion size by measuring it or weighing it:** Don't wait until you feel full to stop eating.
- **Losing a Little Makes a Big Difference:** Break up your weight loss goals into small manageable units of pounds to be lost.
- **Low-Fat Labels Can Be Misleading:** The Nutrition Facts panel on your food is important. You should check it before you purchase or eat a particular food.
- **Eating Out May Be Dangerous:** Eat at home as often as you can.
- **Monitor progress:** Maintaining weight loss is more difficult than losing it.

Key Takeaways

✓ Thinking is a waste of time. Make a plan and do your best to follow it. Remember, nobody is perfect.

✓ A low-carb diet has a proven track record in

helping people lose weight but adherence is the key to success here.

✓ Small dietary modifications (as discussed above) can go a long way in helping you get a healthy body.

✓ Don't go by the reputation of fat in the popular culture. It can be healthy too.

✓ Weight loss is easier than maintaining a healthy weight. When it comes to weight loss, losers are winners.

CHAPTER THREE

Mothers, Daughters, and PCOS

"Anushka, have you finished packing? Pack the stuff too that Nani sent all the way from Kerala."

It was finally time for Anushka to go off on her own. After slogging and slaving away for three full years at SRCC, she had finally achieved what she always wanted—a coveted, high-profile job as an analyst, that too in Blackstone, one of the stalwarts of Wall Street. A driven and ambitious individual, Anushka had always pursued her goals with dogged determinism and like any intelligent dreamer had done it at tremendous personal cost. After graduation, she had moved to Mumbai to live in a dingy single-room flat, powering through multiple internships while simultaneously working on her research, preparing for the opportunity of her lifetime. This inevitably meant long, stressful nights and erratic, unhealthy eating habits— clearly her college diet refused to graduate. But all of that was well worth it now, and why not? Working in New York and living in a company flat was on the top of Anushka's list.

With barely a week to go, all that was left was wrapping up tests and vaccinations. Moving to a whole new country to work for an entirely new company meant various doctors' tests for a whole new range of diseases that frankly only encyclopaedias knew about. One of these included a routine check-up at the gynaecologist. The last time that Anushka had been to one was a long, long time ago, right before college had begun. Now she had put on weight, at an alarming rate. Her Ma thought it could be some hormonal imbalance, something that started with the word poly—

"Ahh, forget it! Those pimples were the miserable after-effect of the giant bars of Toblerone and Mars that had taken over the house when Papa had returned from his Dubai trip. Anyway, best to get over with it, companies and their tests and documents!" said Anushka and went about her work.

***

"Do you mean to tell me that I have cysts on my ovary?" asked Anushka, dazed. She was sitting in the doctor's office, as he examined her test reports. All of this was too much to process for her—a new job, a new country, a new culture, and now a brand new disease to live with. Was this true, had she been living with these cysts for a significant part of her adult life?

What Anushka did not understand, and what the doctor did not articulate, was that Polycystic Ovary Syndrome was a misnomer. Not only was this condition not a disease but also that the cysts referred to follicles, fluid collections that held eggs.

To gain a deeper understanding of this, let's start with Biology for dummies. In a typical menstrual cycle, one of the resting follicles releases an egg from the ovary during the ovulation process. So, PCOS refers to the condition when a woman has a lot of resting follicles that do not ovulate. While most women have 10-15 total resting follicles, women with PCOS may have 10-20 on both ovaries or even more in total.

While the doctor pointed out the more obvious symptoms, irregular periods, oily skin and acne, unexplained weight gain, and sudden facial hair growth (medically termed hirsutism), Anushka didn't understand why this hadn't been detected the last time she was here. To make it even worse, the doctor explained that this had further raised complications and made her susceptible to infertility, type 2 diabetes, cardiovascular problems, and even depression and anxiety. The physical examination results pointed towards PCOS, but only after conducting a pelvic exam, a series of blood tests, and an ultrasound, could the clinic confirm the diagnosis.

Shaken and devastated, Anushka reached home to break this news to her mother. Surprisingly, her mother was not taken aback, anticipating this the first time she suspected the comings of PCOS. She went on to explain to Anushka the tiny details that healthcare practitioners often left out. "Firstly, beta, you have to understand that this is NOT a disease, it cannot hold you back from whatever it is that you want to do with your life. PCOS is simply a hormonal disorder that is extremely common amongst women of reproductive age.

"Fretting and anxiety only add to the stress of the situation. "Clinically, we do know that PCOS is associated with the excessive production of hormones, androgens or testosterone, that are associated with the male sex characteristics and reproduction."

"Ma, how can you stand here and even try to explain to me in cold terms a disease that can put a halt to my life? Do you realize how hard I've worked for this opportunity? It is a once-in-a-lifetime offer. And what about this infertility? I am sure at some point I'd want to bear kids."

With agonizing calmness in her voice, her mother said, "Do you believe this is easy for me, to see my only daughter suffer from a condition that generally passes from generation to generation? To think that I have been skipped to see my child suffer? To think that I did not nag you more when you were in college, did not force you enough to lead a healthier lifestyle and eat well? I should have looked into this more thoroughly when I first suspected it, taken you to more doctors, taken steps of prevention. But that time is gone, and we need first to understand this syndrome—not a disease—to learn how to fight it."

In a voice that was both defeated and angry, Anushka asked, "So what is the next step?"

"Well, the next step is to book an appointment with Dr Pandya. She is the gynaecologist that helped my friend Meera get through this."

At Dr Pandya's they learned that PCOS wasn't easily diagnosed. The reason that it was not detected earlier was that Anushka, being a competitive swimmer in her school days, often used hormonal pills to control her periods. She even attributed her irregular periods to the pills taken then. Unfortunately, explained Dr Pandya, there are no specific symptoms that diagnose it. PCOS is a collection of signs and symptoms that may vary in different women.

"So how will one ever know? I always believed that my acne was simply to do with an unhealthy diet and oily skin."

"I understand that we always tell patients that if we observe two out of these three criteria—irregular menstrual cycles, excess androgen and polycystic ovaries, excessive facial hair and acne—we can confirm our diagnosis."

Anushka sat contemplating how her mother would coax her to avoid consuming dosas, ice creams, hot snacks, packaged foods, et al. How she replaced the cheese with other alternatives and even forced her to go for a run. She never really realized that all those things would matter distinctly in her life.

An enthusiastic biology student in her school days, Anushka knew that androgens were male hormones, so that meant that women with the syndrome showed physical signs of extra androgens, like excess hair growth and high levels of testosterone.

"Why don't you book an appointment for this Friday and we'll schedule you for an ultrasound and a few blood tests?" said the doctor.

Later at home . . .

"Mits, I'm confused; I have no idea how I am going to deal with this and the new job. To top it off, all that Ma does is talk to Reema Masi, who is sitting all the way in Australia. What if this blows up into something even bigger than I can imagine?" complained Anushka. She was speaking with her childhood friend of twenty years, Mitali. She knew Mitali would find a way to soothe her nerves.

"Oh come on, Anushka, quit being so melodramatic. They say 1 in every 5 women in India has PCOS. Even my mom has it. It's just one of those medical syndromes this intrinsically patriarchal universe decided to impose on women. It's nothing that you can't beat."

"Aunty has PCOS, what? When? Didn't she open her restaurant last year? And isn't she expanding with that branch soon? How did she manage all of this alongside the PCOS?"

"Well, you idiot, the same way you'll be able to work at Blackstone and manage it. It's true that you will have to give up your two most adored addictions—Marlboro and sugar—but you would have had to at some point or another. So better now than never."

Anushka and Mitali spoke some more and then hung up.

"Ma, Ma! Are you listening? Get off the phone . . . Guess what Mitali just told me?" Anushka yelled across the room with the renewed hope she once thought could never exist.

"Yes, Anushka, what is it?"

"Did you know that Mitali's mum has PCOS? She had it when Mits was a kid, she even had it when the restaurant was opening, and Mits said it's manageable so long I take care of my eating habits and lifestyle?"

"Of course I did, how else do you think I first detected the symptoms in you? Do you know that Reema Masi also has it, so does Savita bai and a larger number of women around the world? You do not have to worry about it; you can rely on the advice of plenty of people who have experienced the same or worse. Now let's wait until Friday and see what the ultrasound reveals."

It turned out that at the end of the day Anushka did have PCOS; the ultrasound said so loud and clear. This time around, however, it was Ma's turn to worry. Anushka had made peace with the fact, and her conversation with Dr Pandya addressed her significant concerns—treatments can relieve significant symptoms, a healthy diet would go a long way, and oral contraceptives could help with her hormone regulation. In some ways, finding out that she had PCOS was one of the biggest mysteries and reliefs of her life—she had no idea how this happened or why the doctor didn't detect it the last time, but she finally knew why her chin hair was so aggressively persistent.

Dr Pandya also put her on a diet plan that included eating at regular intervals, avoiding simple carbohydrates, and loading up on fibre like whole fruits, beans, and lentils. The doctor also advised her to remain hydrated and avoid saturated fats like cheese, mayonnaise, spreads, and sauces.

But Ma had reason to worry. Anushka had never bothered to lead a healthy lifestyle; she had started smoking when she was 19 and lived off of instant noodles and endless cups of sweet, sweet tea for most of her adult life. Dr Pandya had warned that PCOS almost always translates into insulin resistance and sugar was a big no-no. How was her baby going to manage all on her own? Who would cook for her; make sure she takes her pills, stays off sugar? With such a hectic job, living all by yourself in an unfamiliar country, would Anushka be able to take care of herself? For heaven's sake, she didn't even know that processed food contained hidden sugar? And what about the exercise bit? Who would wake her up once, then twice, then thrice till finally those eyes of hers opened? Who would slap her hand away from grabbing a chocolate granola bar for breakfast instead of sitting down to eat a proper one?

Anushka did not understand her mother's fretting. She could give up sugar and cigarettes, even if that meant not grabbing the last fry but cutting salad for dinner. She was twenty-three years old, she could be trusted with dietary decisions. Blackstone believed her with far, far more than that.

"But beta, they aren't trusting you with somebody's life, na. I trust you with mine."

"Oh come on, Ma, Dr Pandya has left me a list of dos and don'ts, and I'm scheduled to see her in December when I'm back for Christmas. Masi did it too, and she's been working for over 15 years as a PR executive; Mitali's mum is running a successful restaurant, and Savita didi works over 10 hours a day in six houses. These are warriors, and I'm sure with time, I'll become one too! You have to let go of me at some point; I am big enough to take care of myself!"

"Oh great, you're a grown-up now? You haven't even finished the spinach I made you for dinner and you're leaving tomorrow and still not packed. These don't seem to be adult decisions. Now, why don't you go to your room, finish packing, and go off to sleep? You have a long flight tomorrow."

Angry, confused, and scared, Anushka finished packing, took a shower and headed to bed. With full intentions of leaving behind Ma's red sari, the one her mother had hand-embroidered especially for her, Anushka, with an exasperated sigh, flung the little parcel and zipped the suitcase shut. She would miss these fights and debates about life and health and whatnot. These fights meant she had the right suggestion at the end of it all.

It was 4 am. Time to leave. The bags were packed, passport checked, Nani's mathris put in the carry-on bag and kisses met and given. It was only when Anushka went back to her room to grab her watch did she notice the letter with a little diary next to the lamp on the bedside table. It was a letter in the elegant albeit illegible writing of Ma.

Dear Anushka,

It is hard for me to see you as a twenty-three-year-old. The most recent memory I have of you is a ten-year-old licking off her fingers when she finally got her hands on that horrid kalakhatta gola that I always forbid her from eating. The next day you had a terrible stomach ache, but instead of telling me, you marched to Kumar uncle's chemist and defiantly asked for Digene. By evening all was fine, and you were busy eating Maggi while watching Pokémon on TV.

I guess you've always been your person. I've very rarely had to pull you out of trouble or fuss over you—even then you've managed to hold your own. Please understand that I have seen both my mother and my sister go through this; it isn't a biggie, but knowing that it skipped me to plague you makes me feel incredibly guilty. Eating healthy and exercising is a nightmare, take it from a woman who has had two children and diabetes. But make sure that you do it, take your medicine and take the time to cook a meal. Preparing for yourself can be a real adventure sometimes.

Don't let PCOS get the better of you, remember, it is a SYNDROME, not a disease. Live your life exactly the way you had planned it. Become one of those PCOS warriors and send your weary, fretting mother a postcard. Also, remember, PCOS means heightened emotions, so lay-off of the nightly viewing of *This Is Us* for a while.

The diary has a list of easy recipes, a meal plan, diet chart, Dr Pandya's number, nicotine gum, constant reminders to drink water, a few more silly scribbles and a large, large piece of my heart. Take care of it.

Lots and lots of love,
Ma

PS: I'm sorry I scolded you last night. I've packed
a box of sugar-free quinoa brownies for you, to
sample a taste of your new life.

Well, thought Anushka, everything was going to be
okay after all.

Health issues (indeed not every time these issues are
serious problems as some of them just happen to the female
fraternity, say menstruation and menopause) related to our
mothers, daughters, sisters, or simply the womenfolk are
NOT something to ignore or take lightly or joke about.
Because, when ignored and that too for more extended
periods, they may become responsible for a lot of additional
health issues. These addendums take a heavy toll on one's
health resulting in the problems getting transformed
into severe issues. Our society is also one of the primary
factors to be blamed for ignoring or concealing such stuff.
Openness and frank talks are some of the initiatives that are
the need of the hour.

Come out and speak up, ladies, for if you don't speak
up, no one else will.

Fact from figures

Definition: PCOS or Polycystic ovary syndrome is a
condition and a hormonal disorder frequent among women
of reproductive age. Women with PCOS may have unusual
or prolonged menstrual periods or excess male hormone

(androgen) levels. The ovaries may develop numerous small collections of fluid (follicles) and fail to release eggs regularly.

Symptoms:

The symptoms are variable, and a diagnosis is usually made when one experiences the following signs:

a) Irregular menses
b) Excess androgens

Symptoms also include:
•   Weight gain and obesity
•   Hair growth and acne
•   Insulin abnormalities
•   Infertility
•   Heart disease
•   Sleep apnoea

Symptoms of PCOS often develop around the time of the first menstrual period during puberty. Sometimes PCOS develops later, for example, in response to substantial weight gain. PCOS symptoms and signs are typically more severe if you're obese.

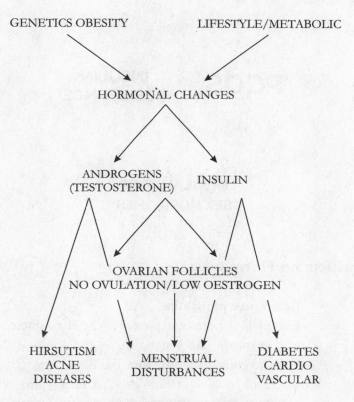

PSYCHOSOCIAL ISSUES: BODY IMAGE,
SELF ESTEEM, DEPRESSION, ANXIETY

Remarkable fact: PCOS affects 1 in 10 women of childbearing age. Such women have a hormonal imbalance and metabolic disorders.

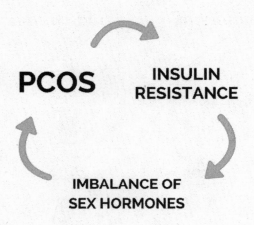

PCOS   INSULIN
RESISTANCE

IMBALANCE OF
SEX HORMONES

Effect on Hormones:

- **Resistance to insulin**

  Insulin is a hormone produced by the pancreas to control the amount of sugar in the blood. It helps to move glucose from the blood into cells, where it's broken down to produce energy. Insulin resistance means the body's tissues are resistant to the effects of insulin. The body, therefore, has to produce extra insulin to compensate. High levels of insulin cause the ovaries to produce too much testosterone, which interferes with the development of the follicles (the sacs in the ovaries where eggs develop) and prevents normal ovulation. Insulin resistance can also lead to weight gain, which can make PCOS symptoms worse, because having excess fat causes the body to produce even more insulin.

- **Hormone imbalance:**

Women with PCOS are found to have an imbalance in certain hormones, including:

  - raised levels of testosterone—a hormone often thought of as a male hormone, although all women usually produce small amounts of it
  - raised levels of luteinising hormone (LH)—this stimulates ovulation but may have an abnormal effect on the ovaries if levels are too high
  - low levels of sex hormone-binding globulin (SHBG)—a protein in the blood, which binds to testosterone and reduces the effect of testosterone
  - raised levels of prolactin (only in some women with PCOS)—a hormone that stimulates the breast glands to produce milk in pregnancy

How to prevent PCOS	How to manage PCOS
Disciplined schedule to manage hormones	Stabilize blood sugar
Avoid skin and hair treatments and cosmetics	Use the right food to combat hirsutism and alopecia
Metformin use	Quit the pill!
Weight loss	Drop your morning coffee!
Infertility treatment	Exercise much to make a difference

Key Takeaways

✓ PCOS refers to the condition when a woman has a lot of resting follicles that do not ovulate.

✓ It is among the leading causes of female infertility.

✓ PCOS increases the risk of developing type 2 diabetes due to insulin resistance.

✓ Irregular periods, multiple small cysts on the ovaries, excess hair on the face and body, acne, or thinning scalp hair may indicate PCOS.

✓ See your doctor, immediately, if you are experiencing such problems for a better prognosis.

CHAPTER FOUR

Salt-y Consequences: Hypertension and Hyper-cholesterol

Lunch hour at C&T Management Consulting meant a cacophony of chatter, laughter, squealing, thumping, and dragging of chairs. However, the one melody that rose above all, the one that dominated, was the powerful resonance of the dabbas. Now, these dabbas by themselves were small meals, but put together they made a feast that could put Punjabi buffets to shame. Our protagonist, Atul Damle, who heads the IT department, has spent most of his life eating simple, fresh, lightly-spiced Maharashtrian food. Before his current employment, Damle had no idea that there was a world of food out there—from spicy fish curries to creamy chicken ones, from hearty rajma to khasta aloo. He found that weirdly enough the company had expanded both his pocket and his palate. Now touching forty-two years, Damle is going to complete his eleventh year with the firm in June. With a receding hairline and expanding waistline, Atul Damle is indeed a happy man.

Recently, though, Damle had reason to be upset. A black cloud had darkened his otherwise sunny existence—Mr Bahl had stopped bringing his dabba from home. Mrs Bahl was indeed a skilled cook—many a lunch had been saved thanks to her tangy green chutney or her deliciously soft puris, and everybody in the office was an ardent fan of her gajar ka halwa. Mrs Bahl left no stone unturned to keep her senior-associate husband well-fed and happy. Unfortunately, fate had something else in store for Mr Bahl: high blood pressure. This meant that the masala and oil had to take a backseat; it was time for Mrs Bahl to master the art of cooking millets and the likes.

What Mr Damle did not understand was how the consumption of home-cooked food could have a hand to play in high BP his colleague had. He wanted his colleague's dabba returned to its former glory.

Well, to begin with, let's examine the meaning of high blood pressure. High blood pressure (HBP or hypertension) is when your blood pressure, the force of the blood flowing through your vessels, is consistently too high. Incidentally, primary hypertension is also called essential hypertension. This kind of hypertension develops over time with no identifiable cause. Most people have this type of high blood pressure. What did this have to do with the diet, Mr Damle wondered? Wasn't eating fresh, home-cooked food and living an active life supposed to keep you healthy and hearty? Not entirely.

Researchers are still unclear what mechanisms cause blood pressure to increase gradually over time. A combination of factors may play a role. Genes are one of them; some people are genetically predisposed to hypertension. Physical changes is another major one.

It's thought that changes in your kidney function due to ageing may upset the body's natural balance of salts and fluid which in turn may cause your body's blood pressure to increase. However, the most common factor and the one you can regulate is your lifestyle. Over time, unhealthy lifestyle choices like poor diet and lack of physical activity can take their toll on the body. Lifestyle choices can lead to problems. Being obese or overweight can increase your risk of hypertension.

When Mr Damle got to know of this, he thought: Ahh, so all that greasy food and those lazy mornings have finally caught up with Mr Bahl. Well, I'm glad I still manage to eat healthy. But the truth was far from that. Mr Damle was a committed bachelor and had enjoyed the comforts of homemade Marathi food until his mother was around. It was almost eight years since her passing, and resignedly, he had taken to convenience foods. This meant that his fridge harboured the 'frozen food family': from pre-cut vegetables to ready-made chapattis, from tinned tomatoes to jarred sauces, he had an excellent collection of ready-to-eat meals, which he was quite proud of. Like any typical bachelor, Damle's go-to finger food was fried fare such as potato nuggets, sausages, and cheese balls, packets and packets of which occupied his freezer shelves.

But soon the unhealthy lifestyle started to show its true colours. An appalling diet combined with the lack of exercise had led to his recent weight-gain, after all, all that the frozen food contained was copious amounts of salt, preservatives, and sodium. Interestingly enough, Mr Damle had not visited a doctor in a while, and with no history of family illness, he found no need for it either.

A few months later, it seemed to Mr Damle that the black cloud was passing; Mrs Bahl had managed to make the best of healthy food. Quinoa had transformed into rich halwa, with dry-fruits scattered all over, paranthas had taken the form of grilled tacos stuffed with a spicy vegetable mixture, and chicken kebabs were now baked not fried, served with hummus instead of her spicy mayo dip. Mr Bahl should not have had reason to complain, yet he continued to fret over lunch on Thursday.

"I can't do this anymore. The doctor says my blood pressure is still rising and refuses to normalize. For heaven's sake, I've tried everything I could—a healthy diet, taking a walk every day, I even went for a morning jog this Sunday. Look at my dabba! All I eat is vegetables and rice," he exclaimed at the lunch table, sprinkling some salt over his boiled broccoli.

"Oh relax, Bahl, you will be fine eventually. Even I went through the same thing. My doctor told me it could be stress and guess what, it was. A year's worth of yoga sessions and weekend baking worked wonders for me. Maybe it's just the long working hours . . . de-stress for a bit and see how it goes?" said Mr Sharma. He happened to be Mr Bahl's boss, holding the position of a senior manager. Only last year he had been diagnosed with hypertension and his doctor had explained that although stress by itself did not cause high BP, other behaviours linked to stress—such as drinking alcohol, overeating, and poor sleeping habits—could cause it. In his case, short-term stress-related spikes had added up over time and put him at risk of developing long-term high blood pressure.

"Believe me, with our kind of work pressure and hectic lifestyle, this had to happen at some point; we aren't twenty anymore. Don't worry, Bahl, it is all part and parcel of life," Mr Sharma said with an air of confidence, dispelling some of Bahl's concern.

"I do hope so, sir. But by the way, how did you figure out you had high blood pressure?"

"Funny story, the doctor had come to my place to conduct a routine check-up on my mother and suggested that I get my blood pressure measured as well, to make sure everything was all right. And well, it wasn't. My BP was well above the normal 120/80."

Unfortunately, if you're looking for a list of symptoms related to high BP, you won't find any. It is because most of the time there are none. It is a myth that people with upper blood pressure experience symptoms like nervousness, sweating, difficulty in facial flushing, or sleeping. The fact is that high blood pressure is a mostly symptomless silent killer. Ignoring it because you believe that a particular symptom or sign will alert you to the problem means taking a fatal risk.

For reasons unknown to him, the conversation between Mr Bahl and Mr Sharma struck a chord with Damle. Reflecting upon his lifestyle and eating habits, Damle thought it best to visit a doctor the first chance he got.

May 23rd would mark the day that Mr Damle learned frozen fruits and vegetables weren't a healthier alternative to pizza and that his body was showing signs of high cholesterol. What had all this got to do with high blood pressure, you ask? And why is cholesterol such a deal-breaker? Doesn't everybody in this day and age struggle to maintain healthy levels of cholesterol?

As Mr Damle learned, men with high total cholesterol are much more likely to develop high blood pressure than men with low total cholesterol. Arteries tend to stiffen and narrow due to cholesterol build-up, and this makes it harder for the heart to pump blood through them. Cholesterol seems to mess up how blood vessels contract and release, which can also affect the pressure needed to push blood through them. Over time, this high pressure damages your arteries and other blood vessels. As a result, they begin to suffer from tears and different types of damage and these tears make a place for the excess of cholesterol; which means that the damage high blood pressure created inside arteries and blood vessels can lead to even more artery narrowing because of high blood cholesterol. In turn, the heart has to work even harder to pump blood, putting excess strain on your heart muscle, leading to heart attacks and other cardiovascular issues.

Studies reveal that high cholesterol and high blood pressure are an unhealthy pair who do their best to mess with your overall health. The doctor explained to Damle that as of now his levels of cholesterol could be controlled which meant blood pressure would remain normal. However, he would have to make some severe changes in his lifestyle to stay healthy.

This gave Damle some clarity, but the one thing that continued to nag him was Mr Bahl's condition. The man had started to exercise and had even switched to healthy eating, giving up all the grease and masala he so dearly loved. All his doctor told him was to book an appointment with the consulting dietician. "I bet she has all the answers you want," he said.

And indeed she did. The secret to regulating both your blood pressure and cholesterol had to do with one unsuspecting ingredient, something no hungry man could imagine—life without salt.

"Salt? Really? Salt."

"Yup, actually salt makes your body retain water. If you overeat, the extra water stored in your body raises your blood pressure. It can be a severe problem if you have high blood pressure. Also, overeating salt may mean that blood pressure medicines, such as diuretics, do not work as well. Therefore reducing the amount of salt you eat is one of the quickest ways to lower your blood pressure. However, it is easier said than done as most of the salt we consume is already in the food we eat."

"So to lower my cholesterol levels, I have to cut down on my salt intake? But I barely eat salt, in fact, I rarely ever add extra salt to my food."

"Well, Mr Damle, could you please give me a quick summary of what you eat on a daily basis?"

"Umm . . . let's see. For breakfast, it is three-minute poha or some cornflakes with milk. Lunch is generally at the office, whatever the canteen serves, pav bhaji or chhole bhature, and of course a little from all of my colleagues' dabbas. Dinner is sabzi and rice and on some days I indulge in some fried food like chicken nuggets or cheese balls."

"This is where the problem lies. Most of the salt we eat every day is 'hidden', which means that it's already in processed foods like biscuits, bread, and breakfast cereals, and prepared ready meals or takeaways. This 'hidden' salt holds around 75% of the salt we eat, only 25% comes from the salt we add while cooking or at the table. The advised intake of salt every day is 6 gms, and from what you're telling me, you are well over the limit."

Mr Damle was aghast.

"Why don't we book an appointment for next week, and I'll draw up a diet chart for you."

Mr Damle nodded and left. But his conversation with the doctor had sparked curiosity in him. Extensive research and a night spent pouring on medical journals revealed that his nutritionist was right after all. He learned that there were primarily three levels of salt intake:

Low: 0.3 gms salt/100 gms
Medium: 0.3-1.5 gms salt/100 gms of food
High: 1.5 gms salt or more/100 gms of food

All of the processed food, canned pulses, and jarred sauces he consumed on a daily basis fell under the medium-high category. Eating excess salt, he learned, lead to an increase in the amount of sodium in the bloodstream and wrecked the delicate balance, reducing the ability of kidneys to remove their water. The result was higher blood pressure due to the extra fluid and extra strain on the blood vessels leading to the kidneys.

It was time for Mr Damle to rethink his dietary choices and re-stock his kitchen. Armed with all this newfound knowledge, he marched happily to the office with the intention of bringing to attention Mr Bahl's culprit: salt. At lunch, Mr Damle explained to him what he had learned at the doctor's office.

"The habit you have of sprinkling extra salt won't do. You can't have cheese-flavoured quinoa; it contains far too much sodium. Ask me, the doctor told me I have high levels of cholesterol, and I've vowed to go off processed foods. No more ready-to-eat rajma for me anymore."

"I'm sorry to hear that, Damle, I know how much you like your snacks and sweets. I guess you'll have to give up all of that as well. You'll have to give up all kinds of fat; cholesterol is very harmful to your body," Mr Bahl chipped in.

It seemed like both of them had learned something new during lunch hour that day.

"Hello Dr Gupta, I have to say you'll be very proud of me," said Damle as soon as he entered his nutritionist's room. "I have completely stopped eating any foods with oil or fat. I've even switched from butter to margarine. I feel like I'm finally on the path to lower cholesterol," he exclaimed proudly.

"But Mr Damle, why would you do that!? Your body needs good cholesterol to function. This is not a solution. Are you familiar with the concept of cholesterol?"

"Well, yes, of course. It is an unnecessary plaque or fat that our body stores when we eat unhealthy food, right?"

"Ahh, nope. Although that is what most people believe to be true. Cholesterol is a type of fat in your blood. Your cells need cholesterol, and your body makes all you need. But you also get cholesterol from the food you eat. For decades we've been told that dietary cholesterol is bad and that it clogs your arteries. The fact is that this portrayal of cholesterol as an artery-clogging fat is false. Cholesterol makes key hormones and is essential for brain and nerve function. Your liver makes about three-quarters of the body's cholesterol—this is important stuff!"

"So, a good kind of cholesterol exists?"

"Yes, of course! There are two kinds of cholesterol. Low-density lipoprotein (LDL) is often called bad cholesterol. It carries cholesterol to your arteries. If your levels of LDL cholesterol are too high, it can build up on the walls of your arteries, also called cholesterol plaque. This plaque can narrow your arteries, limit your blood flow, and raise your risk of blood clots.

"The other kind, the right type is High-density lipoprotein (HDL). It helps return LDL cholesterol to your liver to be removed from your body. This helps prevent cholesterol plaque from building up in your arteries.

"So you see, not all cholesterol is wrong."

"Doctor, what foods help in increasing the HDL levels?"

"Well, an ideal HDL level is 60 milligrams/decilitre (mg/dL) or above. Such heart-healthy fats or unsaturated fats are found in olive oil, nuts, whole grains, legumes and beans, fatty fish and of course exercise counts too. It is also important to view your genetic profile, not all cholesterol is generated by unhealthy food."

"Also, I'm scared that all of this puts me at heart risk. In case I'm unable to regulate cholesterol levels, does that mean surgery for me?"

"Of course not, Mr Damle, that's the last resort. Unless you're at high risk of heart problems, have a worrisome family history, particularly of early heart attack and death, you won't need cholesterol-lowering drugs or surgery. And my last piece of advice: stay off any food item that says no-fat or low-fat; it is more than likely to be processed food that contains high amounts of sugar."

Mr Damle nodded.

"Well, I'll see you next week, then?"

And so, our dear Mr Damle followed Dr Gupta's diet chart, monitored his daily salt intake, stayed off margarine, enjoyed ghee-slathered paranthas once in a while, and led a happy, happy life completing twenty-five successful years at C&T Management Consulting. Thanks to Dr Gupta, even Mr Bahl managed to lower his blood pressure. And yes, Damle continued to stave off of Mr Bahl's dabba for the rest of his lunch hours; he was a creature of habit after all.

Unfortunately, unlike Mr Damle and Mr Bahl, not everybody gets their happy ending. In this age of convenience foods, we often get too occupied with our careers and forget to take care of ourselves. Cooking for yourself can be an exciting experience. From sitting down and sharing meals with our family and friends, we've moved to the grab-and-go generation. Processed food has flooded the market. Unfortunately, convenience foods are not all that convenient for your health. High amounts of hidden sugar, sodium, and preservatives can have damaging consequences in the future, and so it is time we think more about the food we eat. Living Mr Damle's life might be achievable after all.

Many around us believe that if you eat home-cooked food items, where these food items be anything, you will live long and healthy! Because homemade delicacies ought to be healthy, always. This stereotype must be shown the door, once and for all, for the betterment of the society. So, let's expand the phrase 'any home-cooked food item' and its relationship with a 'long and healthy life.' And by expansion, I mean development focused on one particular word—any.

In the busy and exhaustive schedules of our day-to-day lives, we ignore the most important factor that directly determines our health condition: the food we consume. Are home-cooked food items always healthy for everyone? Ask this question to yourself every time you prepare your mind to destroy anything that features as 'bad for health' in medical terms. If you are a formally working person, who physically & mentally wears down itself during office hours day after day; take a break and look around yourself. More than half of your colleagues, departmental heads, supervisors, managers, and subordinates who are living like you, i.e. eating homemade food items during lunch, have unknowingly developed health complications they're not even aware of by now.

The human body is the most complex working machine that functions almost perfectly. It gives warning signs about any abnormality within it, many of which are bluntly ignored. The health complication developments I mentioned earlier are the most common ones that are visible in almost every random person. These are:

- Hypertension
- High blood pressure
- High levels of cholesterol

Most apparent reasons for the occurrence of the above three are:

- Unhealthy lifestyle
- Poor diet plan
- Lack of adequate physical activities/exercises

Mathematically, the number of unknown variables requires at least those many numbers of equations for obtaining the solution. Here for three problems, we have three answers. But life is not some algebraic mumbo-jumbo or a child's play of mere statistics. It's more than that; so we have to deal with it likewise.

Here are a few handy tips for a healthy heart:
✓ Ditch excess salt
✓ Get up and move
✓ Don't smoke

- ✓ Keep your weight in check
- ✓ Add more fibres to your diet
- ✓ Show the door to saturated fats
- ✓ Eat at least 5 portions of a variety of fruit and vegetables a day
- ✓ Keep an eye on food labels for unwanted ingredients
- ✓ Keep alcohol intake to zero to minimum

Did You Know?

For Breakfast		
Day 1		
What I have	What Granny had	What went wrong
Muesli and toast with butter	Homemade porridge	The high salt content in bread and hidden salt in muesli
Day 2		
What I have	What Granny had	What went wrong
Cheese Sandwich and Juice (Tetra Pak)	Gobi parantha and homemade curd	Cheese is laden with sodium and packaged juice has emulsifiers and stabilisers
For Snacks		
What I have	What Granny had	What went wrong
Cookie with creamy coffee	Homemade tea with puffed rice	A cookie-based product contains high salt. Machine coffee made from creamer has chemicals and synthetic flavouring agents

For Lunch		
What I have	What Granny had	What went wrong
6-inch Subway with soup	Dal-rice made at home with green vegetables	Subway bread and sauces have high sodium content, veggies used are in brine (salt solution). Soup is made from soup cubes which are again high on salt and artificial flavours
Evening go-to snack		
What I have	What Granny had	What went wrong
Croissant with green tea	Tea with homemade besan pakoda	Croissant being a bakery product has white flour and a lot of salt whereas homemade pakoda has very limited salt
Evening go-to snack		
What I have	What Granny had	What went wrong
Order biryani	Two chapattis with aloo sabzi	Biryani cooked in stores outside have more salt
Instant foods like rajma, paneer, or noodles	Dal, chapatti, and rice	All instant and ready-to-eat foods have higher salt to increase shelf-life

Table Highlights:

The table clearly points out choosing food over what my grandmother ate, I have added an excess of salt load to my food as I have picked up easy-to-eat food items which are mostly packaged. It has increased the sodium content in food.

Fact 1: Normal person's sodium requirement is less than 6 grams of salt.

Fact 2: Most urban working Indians eat up to three times of the recommended norms.

How do I decrease my sodium intake:

1. Don't eat from a box, tin, canned Tetra Pak or a bottle.
2. Increase intake of fibre from fresh fruits and veggies to counter higher salt intake.
3. Drink more water. Do not choose coffee. Choose water to remain hydrated.
4. Munch on nuts (unsalted), paneer, homemade chiwra.
5. Replace cakes and desserts with home-made halwa and kheer.
6. Bakery products are a big no! (bread, cookies, buns, ready-to-eats)
7. Flavour your food with home-made dips made of yoghurt, mint instead of spreads and mayonnaise.

NOTES:

....

....

....

....

CHAPTER FIVE

Eat, Beat, and Survive

When I was young, childhood was carefree. Our days were spent in learning, playing, helping mum at home and running small errands. I remember how Dad would always tell me to do my share of jobs for the house, fill the cooler with water in the evening, buy bread, milk, and eggs for the next morning from the milk vendor around the corner, ensure the main door was locked, and the garbage removed before bedtime.

All this and more became part of my learning to live a normal life: simple rules to learn basic cooking, polish your own shoes, and iron your own uniform. There was pride and value attached to simplicity. Vacations were far and few and most of our summer holidays were limited to visiting our relatives. Treats on special occasions were limited to halwa puri and kheer. Life was blissful.

That was also the time when disease was not on our minds and the only sickness we caught was an odd fever or flu or a stomach upset. Our parents were worried about us breaking a limb while running on the terrace or climbing a tree.

Cut to present times: Ragini, a seventeen-year-old girl, has been diagnosed with Lymphoma, a type of cancer that spreads to various body tissues. While the lymph system typically protects your body, lymph cells called lymphocytes can become cancerous. Lymphomas can affect any portion of the lymphatic system, including, bone marrow, spleen, tonsils, and lymph nodes. Lymphomas are divided into two categories: Hodgkin's lymphoma and non-Hodgkin's lymphoma.

Ragini is sitting in the chemotherapy recliner and waiting for her session to start. She has not eaten breakfast for fear of throwing up. She is suffering from fear of the therapy, the pain, the after effects while battling hunger at the same time.

CANCER, a word that was alien to us just fifty years back, seems to have touched most lives. We all know of somebody from our family or friends who is struggling with this disease, which sounds both scary and mysterious. Cancer is of so many types with such a complex prognosis that each person who gets cancer has a unique journey of cancer treatment.

A large part of cancer management lies in cancer prevention: if we can eliminate things or agent capable of causing cancer (called carcinogens)—toxic chemicals, heavy metals, plastics, radiation, etc., and include anti-cancer elements such as deep breathing, aerobic exercises, colourful fruits and vegetables, spices and flavourful herbs—we can hope to live a cancer-free life.

What really is Cancer?

A question that has a debatable answer is what is cancer? And what has really happened to the environment? Though the entire thought has been receiving attention from scientists, policymakers, and even the public but we all shall remain curious as the disease or condition called cancer takes years to develop an outbreak into lives.

But what really is cancer? It's a disease with several clinical conditions, symptoms, and variable range of severity. The processes occurring in cancer at the cellular level are all common. The cellular processes may or may not lead to the disease but it may help us narrow down on the compounds from the environment that may lead to cancer.

Many suggest that all forms of cancer are an outcome of a single type of cell that is being reproduced in a disordered way. This production happens at an abnormally fast pace and leads to a condition called cancer. There are multiple environmental factors that may be associated with cancer or its cause. Following are the possibilities:

1. DNA-damaging chemicals. These carry information for cells to reproduce.
2. Cell reproduction-regulating chemicals.
3. Epigenetic modification or reversible changes inducing chemicals.
4. Infectious agents and viruses.
5. Immune system harming agents.

It is difficult for scientists to consider large groups of people and understand what amount of an agent is actually causing cancer. But recent research lays the foundation of whatever we know about the environment and cancer.

The causes of cancer can be broadly categorized into the following:

1. Behavioural factors: includes smoking, diets.
2. Occupational factors: work histories, exposure to different kinds of chemicals.

Cancer is the second leading cause of death globally and was responsible for an estimated 9.6 million deaths in 2018. Globally, about 1 in 6 deaths is due to cancer. Have a look into the numbers? About 16% of people die from cancer! Astonishing numbers? But all true. Surprisingly, about 70% of all deaths from cancer occur in low- and middle-income countries.

In 2018, the top 5 types of cancer that killed men were lung, liver, stomach, colorectal, and prostate, reports WHO. Around 1/3rd of deaths from cancer are due to the 5 leading behavioural and dietary risks: high body mass index, low fruit and vegetable intake, lack of physical activity, tobacco use, and alcohol use. Tobacco use is the most important risk factor for cancer and is responsible for approximately 22% of cancer deaths.

The 5 most common types of cancers that kill women are breast, lung, colorectal, cervical, and stomach.

Cancer may be solid or metastatic. A solid cancer is a malignancy that forms a discrete tumour mass and is usually limited to a certain body organ or part such as cancer of breast, prostate, colorectal, kidney, etc.

Metastatic cancer is one in which the cancer cells can spread locally by moving into nearby normal tissue. Cancer can also spread regionally, to nearby lymph nodes, tissues, or organs. And it can spread to distant parts of the body. For many types of cancer, it is also called stage IV (four) cancer such as leukaemia, which may diffusely infiltrate a tissue without forming a mass. The process by which cancer cells spread to other parts of the body is called metastasis.

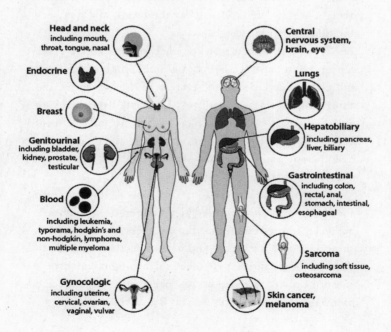

Common Cancers in Men and Women

The story:

I have met many young men and women battling cancer during my practice. I am always amazed to see their will to fight through the thick and thin of life and disease conditions. Their persona is so addictive that we all start drawing inspiration from them. I am fortunate to have met a man like this who was diagnosed with cancer and was undergoing treatment. He was asked to take regular treatment and chemotherapy, as generally advised to a cancer patient. He was treated entirely from disease and was living a healthy life until one day the lymphoma was back and this time with a vengeance.

This young man was shattered. The pain of undergoing cancer treatment once before and imbibing body changes and physical and mental and emotional changes always has a huge impact on personal lives. The same happened with this young man. He lost complete faith in medical treatment and declined all ways and means of treatment including radiotherapy and chemotherapy. He knew that this would not treat cancer. He was sure this time.

This young man went to the US, only to stay and learn about Gerson's Therapy. He did not undergo any treatment but solely learned about this therapy. Gerson's Therapy is a specialized diet for cancer and looks into the treatment of all forms of the disease. He relied on it to fight with cancer and not on any medication. His belief in the therapy and following of the protocols was his line of treatment.

What shook him was the fact that only if he had known earlier, then he could have avoided cancer. Knowing that nutrition is the most significant form of saviour from cancer and having a scheduled diet can be a big boon. He focused on food and food until he got better.

Dr Gerson's therapeutic techniques involved having each patient use an integrated set of particular healthcare methods and management, including focussing on the following:

a) Salt and water management through sodium (Na) mineral restriction and potassium (K) mineral supplementation.

b) Superabundant intake (higher alimentation) of both macronutrients and micronutrients through the regular hourly preparation of drinking of raw, organically grown fruits and vegetable juices.

c) Extreme limitation of fats consumed in foods.

d) Temporary protein restriction through a basically vegan diet.

e) Natural supplemental thyroid administration.

f) Production of bile by the liver by means of frequent self-administered coffee enemas.

Gerson's Therapy is a series of harmonics and cohesive medical treatments that have cured many individual cases of advanced cancer.

Nowadays people have a common concern if the environment they live in may increase their risk of cancer. And, sadly we are all out of opinions and answers for this concern. Therefore, it is as important to understand if cancer in any way is associated with the risk of developing cancer.

It is not easy to answer this question for several reasons, the most prominent of which is that the majority of cancers take years, or even decades, to develop. Scientists rarely have the opportunity to make a large number of people measure the amount of a specific pollutant they are exposed to, and then follow them over time to see if they develop cancer.

Everyday things that increase cancer risks:

	Carcinogen/ Mutagen	Correction/ Solution
Eating Red Meat/ Charred Meat	DNA altering chemicals	Replace with vegetarian protein such as vegetables, legumes, beans.
Plastic Water Bottles	Chemicals like BPA, a synthetic hormone	Use glass, steel bottles.
Being Sedentary	10-20% increase in colon, endometrial, and lung cancer	Mild exercises Move every 30 minutes.
Wearing Deodorants	Aluminium compounds— change oestrogen receptors	Wear a natural, plant-based perfume.

	Carcinogen/ Mutagen	Correction/ Solution
Microwave Popcorn	Diacetyl butter flavouring Bladder cancer	Make popcorn from plain corn and add herbs to flavour.
Make-up and skincare	Parabens absorbed by skin—breast cancer	Stay natural; use minimal makeup.
Working night shift/being late at night	Leads to melatonin suppression	Maintain regular and respectable body clocks.
Cleaning products (fabric softeners, dishwashing liquids, disinfectants)	Formaldehyde	Use plain soap and dilute acid for cleaning.
Styrofoam cups and plates	Styrene that is used to make these cups and plates	Don't use Styrofoam for hot liquids. Use ceramic, glass, or steel.

Cancer and Nutrition:

Nutrition and food science have each enhanced the development of an abundant, nutritious, and safe food supply. A healthy diet should contain all of the required nutrients and sufficient calories to balance energy expenditure and provide for growth and maintenance throughout the life cycle.

Dietary factors are associated with 5 of the 10 leading causes of death, including coronary heart disease, certain types of cancer, stroke, noninsulin-dependent diabetes mellitus, and atherosclerosis. Each stage of the life cycle has specific nutrient needs. Throughout infancy, childhood, and adolescence, nutrients are required to meet the growth processes as well as cognitive function. During pregnancy, nutrients are required for both mother and developing infant needs. Adult nutrition focuses on tissue maintenance, nutrient and energy needs, and disease prevention. As the population of elderly increase in number, nutritional needs must be met to minimize certain disease states and assure the quality of life. Nutrition associated health risks have been identified for coronary heart disease, cancer, and diabetes mellitus. Recommendations for each include a decrease in dietary fat, awareness of caloric intake, and enhancement of nutrient density including an increase in fruit and vegetables. These recommendations also impact obesity and diminish the compounding of other disease states affected by excessive body weight. Calcium intake at early ages affects the development of bone density and the manifestation of osteoporosis.

Current gaps in knowledge are also identified that could improve health. Numerous nutrients are being examined for their regulation of specific gene expressions and in the processes of transcription and translation. To offer food products with greater nutrient density or improved functional health ingredients, modification of existing foods is needed to assure an improved diet. Policies to improve health requires the integration of nutrition needs with economic growth and development, agriculture and food production, processing, marketing, health care and education, and include changing lifestyle and food choices.

Increased research support is required to achieve national health goals with an emphasis on nutrition and food sciences. Education methods must be improved to better inform consumers, to encourage food producers and manufacturers to produce healthier foods, to assure training of future professionals and to provide legislators with the basis to make informed decisions. A decrease in the occurrence and duration of chronic disease should diminish the cost of healthcare and allow these resources to further benefit the nation. International concerns about undernutrition include 780 million people who are malnourished, lacking sufficient food to meet their basic nutritional needs for protein and energy and 2 billion people who subsist on diets lacking essential nutrients needed for growth, development, and physiological maintenance. National concerns about undernutrition exist based on incomplete data identified by indices of hunger and characterized by an increased demand for food assistance for women, children, and the elderly.

Good Nutrition During Cancer Treatment

Cancer treatment can place a lot of nutritional demand on your body. It is important to try to consistently consume a healthy diet and to drink nourishing beverages. The main nutritional goals during this time are to maintain a healthy weight and eat healthy foods that supply your body with calories and nutrients for energy, repair, recovery, and healing. A healthful eating pattern includes plenty of vegetables and fruit, moderate amounts of whole grains, and plant protein sources like nuts, beans, lentils, tofu, and tempeh, along with modest portions of fish, poultry, lean meats, and non-fat or low-fat dairy foods.

Treatment Side-Effects That Can Impact Nutritional Well-Being

Side-effects of cancer therapy may affect your eating habits and nutritional status. Here are some suggestions for managing common eating difficulties during and after treatment.

Changes in Appetite and Unwanted Weight Loss

Loss of appetite is common in people with cancer and can lead to weight loss and undernutrition. Poor nutrition can slow the body's ability to heal. Severe malnutrition can interfere with the proper functioning of the heart, liver, kidneys, and immune system. Try these ideas for improving your appetite and maintaining calorie and protein intake during cancer treatment:

- Eat five or six smaller meals per day.
- Eat the largest meal when you are the hungriest.
- Start with high-protein foods while your appetite is strongest.

- Keep favourite high-calorie foods and beverages within easy reach.
- Try to be as physically active as you are able to be to help stimulate your appetite.
- Enlist the help of your loved ones and caregivers to help with purchasing and preparing food.

Nausea and Vomiting

Nausea and vomiting can be caused by chemotherapy or from radiation therapy to the stomach, abdomen, or brain. Being nauseated or vomiting because of cancer treatment can make it difficult for a person to eat and drink. Try these ideas for managing nausea and vomiting:

- Eat small amounts of food more often.
- Small portions of meals and snacks are often easier to tolerate than large.
- Eating foods and sipping on clear liquids at room temperature or cooler may be easier to tolerate.
- Avoid high-fat, greasy, spicy, or overly sweet foods.
- Avoid foods with strong odours.
- Sip on beverages between meals rather than with meals.
- Eat sitting up and keep head raised for about an hour after eating.
- In case of vomiting, avoid eating or drinking until vomiting is controlled—then try sipping on small amounts of clear liquids such as cranberry juice or broth.

- Nibbling on plain foods such as an orange, plain cookies, or crackers may also help.
- Take anti-nausea medicine as prescribed.

Fatigue

Fatigue is the most common side-effect for those diagnosed with cancer. It can be related to the cancer itself or can be one of the effects of cancer treatment. Eating regularly and being as physically active as you are able to be may help relieve your fatigue and enhance your mood.

In certain situations, your doctor may prescribe a medication to help improve your appetite. Try to drink plenty of fluids. Being dehydrated can make fatigue worse.

Try these ideas for managing fatigue:
- Temporarily rely on ready-to-eat foods like frozen dinners, fruits, and vegetables.
- Prepare food when you feel your best and freeze leftovers in meal-size portions.
- Try to drink plenty of fluids. Being dehydrated can make fatigue worse. Aim for at least 8-10 cups of hydrating fluid each day unless advised to restrict fluids for another medical condition. Hydrating fluids include water, clear juices, sports drinks, broth, or weak tea.
- Accept help with meals from friends and family members.

Bowel Changes: Diarrhoea and Constipation

Diarrhoea can be caused by cancer itself, certain chemotherapy agents and medicines, or because of radiation therapy to the abdomen and pelvis. Diarrhoea is having frequent and loose watery stools.

Try these ideas for managing this:
- Drink plenty of liquids such as water, clear juices, sports drinks, broth, weak tea, or oral rehydration solutions (available over-the-counter at most pharmacies).
- Eat small amounts of soft, bland foods. Consider a diet that consists of water-soluble fibre-containing foods such as bananas, white rice, applesauce, and white toast.
- Decrease intake of high fibre foods during this time. These include foods containing nuts and seeds, raw vegetables and fruits, and whole grain breads and cereals.
- Eat small amounts of food throughout the day rather than fewer large meals.
- Take anti-diarrhoea medicine as prescribed.

Constipation can be a symptom of cancer itself or it can be caused by medicines used to treat cancer or manage pain. Constipation is when bowels do not move regularly and when stools become hard and difficult to pass. Try these ideas for managing constipation:

- Drink more healthy beverages to help keep your digestive system moving, especially water, prune juice, warm juices, decaffeinated teas, and hot lemonade.
- Increase intake of high fibre foods such as whole grains, fresh and cooked vegetables, fresh and dried fruits, and foods containing peels, nuts, and seeds.
- Work with your healthcare team to set up an individualized bowel regimen. This program may include stool softeners and gentle, non-habit forming laxatives.
- Increase your physical activity, as you are able to, such as taking a walk or doing limited exercise every day.

Changes in Taste and Smell

Changes in taste and reactions to smells are common problems that can happen while undergoing and recovering from cancer treatment. These changes can affect your desire to eat.

Try these ideas for managing taste and smell changes:
- Choose foods that appeal to you. Often, moist and naturally sweet foods such as frozen melon balls, grapes, or oranges work well. Some find tart foods and beverages appealing.
- Try eating cooler temperature foods, rather than hotter temperature foods, as they have less aroma and taste.
- Try marinades and spices to mask strange tastes.

Brush your teeth and tongue and rinse your mouth regularly, especially before eating.

- Rinse your mouth several times a day with 1 to 2 ounces of homemade salt and baking soda solution (one quart of water combined with one teaspoon of salt and one teaspoon of baking soda) or an alcohol-free mouth rinse.

Sore Mouth or Throat

A common side effect of certain chemotherapy agents or radiation therapy to the mouth and throat is an inflammation of the mucus membranes that line the mouth and throat. This condition is called mucositis and it can make it difficult to eat and swallow.

Try these ideas for managing a sore mouth or throat:

- Eat soft, moist foods with extra sauces, dressings, or gravies.
- Avoid dry, coarse, or rough foods.
- Avoid alcohol, citrus, caffeine, vinegar, spicy foods, and acidic foods (like tomatoes).
- Experiment with temperatures of foods (warm, cool, or icy) to find which temperature is the most soothing.
- Drink plenty of fluids. Focus on warm or cool milk-based beverages, non-acidic fruit drinks (diluted if necessary) and broth-based soups.
- Rinse your mouth several times a day with 1 to 2 ounces of homemade salt and baking soda solution

(200 ml of water combined with one teaspoon of salt and one teaspoon of baking soda). Sip, swish, and then spit the solution to rinse and clean your mouth. Do not swallow.

Unwanted Weight Gain
Weight gain can occur during or after treatment for hormone-sensitive cancers such as breast or prostate cancers. Inactivity can also cause weight gain. In addition, medicines such as steroids used as a part of some cancer treatments can contribute to increased weight.

Try these ideas for managing unwanted weight gain:
- Try to focus on foods naturally low in calories and high in fibre to help you feel full, such as vegetables, fruits, whole grains, and beans. Include small amounts of higher-calorie foods that you enjoy most, and be sure to savour them for the most satisfaction.
- Pay attention to portion sizes and fill most of your plate with lower-calorie plant foods. Eat only when you are physically hungry.
- Try to get regular physical activity to help reduce fatigue, control weight gain, and improve mood.

Low White Blood Cell Counts and Infection
Cancer and cancer treatment can weaken the immune system and increase the risk of infection. White blood

cells are an essential part of the body's defence against infection because they attack and destroy germs after they enter the body. The risk of infection increases as the number of white blood cells decreases as the result of some cancer treatments. This condition is called Neutropenia. If you develop neutropenia it is very important to protect yourself against infection. Contact your healthcare team right away if you think an infection is developing.

The following may be signs of infection:
- A temperature greater than 100.5° F.
- Fever.
- Shaking, chills.
- Swelling or redness of any part of the body.

If you experience a period of time when your white blood cell counts are low, eat a 'safe food' diet to avoid harmful bacteria and food-borne illnesses. Follow these 'safe food'/neutropenic suggestions when your white blood cell counts are low:
- Do not eat raw or undercooked animal products, including meat, pork, poultry, eggs, and fish.
- Wash all fresh fruits and vegetables.
- Avoid eating foods from salad bars or eating pre-cut fruits.
- Do not drink untested well water or water directly from lakes, rivers, streams, or springs. If using filtered water, change the filter regularly.

Food Safety Tips

These food safety tips are especially important for people undergoing and recovering from cancer treatment:

1. Wash hands frequently. Use plenty of soap and hot, running water for at least twenty seconds. Use hand sanitizer for cleaning hands when soap and water are not available. Wash or sanitize hands:
    *   After using the restroom.
    *   Before eating.
    *   Before and after each step of food preparation.
    *   After handling garbage.
    *   After touching pets.
    *   After sweeping the floor or wiping down the counters.
2. Keep cutting boards, countertops, and utensils thoroughly cleaned. Change, launder, and discard sponges and dishtowels often.
3. Separate and do not cross-contaminate.
4. Keep raw meat, poultry, seafood, and eggs away from ready-to-eat foods.
5. Cook food thoroughly at proper temperatures. Use a food thermometer to make sure foods are safely cooked.
6. Properly wrap and refrigerate foods promptly. Refrigerate or freeze leftover foods within one hour to limit the growth of bacteria.

7. Set the refrigerator between 34° F and 40° F. Keep the freezer set to 0–2° F or below.
8. Pay attention to food product expiration dates. If in doubt, throw it out.

Cancer and Nutrition
Connecting the dots

The link between cancer and diet is just as mysterious as the disease itself. Research has pointed toward certain foods and nutrients that may help prevent—or, conversely, contribute to—certain types of cancer.

While there are many factors you can't change that increase your cancer risks, such as genetics and environment, there are others you can control. In fact, estimates suggest that less than 30% of a person's lifetime risk of getting cancer results from uncontrollable factors. The rest you have the power to change, including your diet.

Keep in mind that most research only points to associations between diet and cancer, and not necessarily a cause-and-effect relationship. "It is not 100% certain that consuming more or less of certain foods or nutrients will guarantee cancer protection," says Dr Edward Giovannucci of Harvard's TH Chan School of Public Health. "But science has found that certain dietary habits tend to have a greater influence." Here is a look at four areas that stand out.

1. **Processed and red meat**

   Processed meat is any meat that has been smoked or fermented or includes added salt and nitrites to enhance flavour. The connection between processed meat and cancer is consistent. For instance, about 30 prospective studies of colorectal cancer—the third most diagnosed cancer in men—found that eating around 50 grams a day of processed meat is associated with about a 20% increase in colorectal cancer risk. The risk factors are similar to red meat, too. The exact mechanism is unclear, but it may be related to the added nitrates in processed meat and the heme iron inherently found in red meat.

2. **Antioxidants**

   Antioxidants, no doubt, are important for cancer prevention, as they help neutralize free radicals that can damage cells. But the larger question is whether taking more through your diet or supplements further reduces your risk.

   "So far the research to support the more-is-better approach has not been impressive," says Dr Walter Willett of the TH Chan School of Public Health. "We don't yet know how long you would need to take extra antioxidants for a benefit to be seen," he says. "Some cancers develop over many decades, and you may need to increase dietary antioxidants in your early years to see a benefit."

   Still, it's important to consume foods high in antioxidants, since they offer other benefits, too, like improved cardiovascular health. Do not target individual antioxidants, but instead aim for a diet that includes a variety of high-antioxidant foods. Focus on bright colours, such as dark green, orange, purple, and red fruits and vegetables—for instance, spinach, carrots, and tomatoes.

3. **Glycaemic index**

Carbohydrates have a Jekyll-and-Hyde role with cancer: they can be good or bad depending on the source. Glycaemic index (GI), a measure of how fast carbohydrates turn into sugar in the blood, helps us tell the good from the bad.

A study of 3,100 people, presented at the 2016 Experimental Biology forum, found that consuming foods with a high GI (70 or higher on the 100-point GI scale) was associated with an 88% greater risk for prostate cancer. High-GI items include sugar-sweetened soft drinks, fruit juices, and processed foods like pizza.

On the flip side, eating lower-GI foods like legumes (beans, lentils, and peas) was linked with a 32% lower risk of both prostate and colorectal cancers. Another study, published in March 2015 in *Cancer Epidemiology, Biomarkers & Prevention*, linked a high-GI diet with lung cancer, the second most common cancer among men. The study showed an almost 50% increase in risk among people with the highest GI diet compared with those with the lowest.

Low- and medium-GI foods rank from 0 to 69 on the GI scale.

4. **Calcium**

Some evidence suggests higher calcium intake can lower the risk for cancer, especially colorectal cancer. Researchers believe calcium binds to bile acids and fatty acids in the gastrointestinal tract. This acts as a shield to protect cells from the damaging stomach acids.

However, other research has shown that extra calcium—2,000 milligrams (mg) or more per day—may be linked to a higher risk of prostate cancer. Your best bet is to keep your daily calcium intake to 500 mg to 1,000 mg per day, either from food like dairy products, nuts, millets, or supplements.

5. **Weight gain and cancer**

Another way to look at diet's role in cancer prevention is in terms of weight management. Modifying your diet can keep your weight under control, which offers even more protection.

A 2014 study in the journal *The Lancet* found that a higher body mass index increases the risk of developing some of the most common cancers. Scientists discovered that among five million people studied, a gain of 34 pounds was linked with a 10% or higher risk for colon, gallbladder, kidney, and liver cancers. The connection? Experts say body fat produces hormones and inflammatory proteins that can promote tumour cell growth.

Burger and Dal Theory

This theory must have produced some desirable saliva in your mouth. However, how would you like to know that one-time replacement of Burger meal to Dal meal can improve your chances of precaution against cancer by 0.10%? Here, freshness is the secondary point; a burger contains an excessive amount of iron supplements which promotes the formation of a tumour and metastasizes into colorectal cancer. These two supplements are ferric citrate and ferric EDTA.

The high or low amount of these two iron supplements in not only burgers but in any cuisine can stimulate as a risk factor for cancer.

Dal has always been in the good books of moms and why not? From mild fever to cancer risk, dal has turned out to be a precautious element. Pulses are low fat and rich protein nutritional eatables contributing as an anticancer ingredient for a long time now.

Since the world has positioned its taste buds to the high fat, animal protein, and high carbohydrate food, the worth of contradicted food elements like pulses, Indian spices, fruits, beans, and Ayurvedic teas has become restricted to diet theories only. This is the right time to switch from risky food factors like junk to cancer-fighting food factors.

How was the food at home anti-cancerous food?

The food at home surely has love; however, what it mainly has is an adequate amount of healthy food ingredients. Cancer Research has concluded—

- Cruciferous vegetables like broccoli, cauliflower, and Brussels sprouts contain nutritious elements like crambene and glucosinolate which distort the production of abnormal cells in the stomach, mouth, breast, skin, and even oesophagus.
- Do you remember that irresistible smell of garlic which makes the food smell enormously delicious? Yes, this small food ingredient, which is used almost every day, helps to prohibit the formation of any tumour in the human body.
- Tea is again one of the most likely drinks to be consumed at least two times a day. The tea elements fight against cancer within your body. Doctors mention that if there is any present cancerous tumour within the human body, tea helps to reduce the size of a tumour and fortunately, can reduce it to zero in the long run.
- A tomato is a fruit which works as an important element for gravy. It is an anti-cancerous substance. These red beauties contain lycopene which attacks the cell with incompatible growth and protects the well-built cells from damage.

Likewise, whole grain, fruit meals, carrots, and bean-based meals work as unpaid and proven medications for protection against cancer.

Phytochemicals and their food sources in cancer prevention:

Phytochemical in Food	Food Sources	Possible Cancer Benefits	Consumption Ideas
Flavonoids	Apples, berries, cherries, citrus fruits, plums, whole grain, nuts	Helps prevents cancers such as oral, breast, lung, thyroid, prostate, colon, leukaemia	Have raw fruits 3 or more times a day and consume only whole grain, stay away from refined flour or grain
Ally Sulphides	Onions, garlic, leeks, ginger	May reduce the risk of certain cancers such as skin, prostate, and liver	Eat raw and use for seasoning and cooking

Phytochemical in Food	Food Sources	Possible Cancer Benefits	Consumption Ideas
Catechins	Flavoured teas, masala teas, fresh green tea (with leaves)	May reduce the risk of certain cancers such as colon, lung, liver, and lymphoma	Drink your homemade tea, replace coffee with tea
Carotenoids (lutein, b-carotene, lycopene)	Deeply coloured fruits and vegetables such as tomatoes, sweet potatoes, peppers, potatoes, and spinach	Helps prevents cancers such as prostate, breast, lungs and blood cancer	Just add them to all your meals, blend into a thick juice, eat as cooked vegetables, make salads, stuff in millets to make chapattis
Indoles	Broccoli, cauliflower, cabbage, turnips and Brussels sprouts	May reduce the risk of certain cancers such as breast and colon	Just add them to all your meals, blend into a thick juice, eat as cooked vegetables, make a salad, stuff in millets to make chapattis

Phytochemical in Food	Food Sources	Possible Cancer Benefits	Consumption Ideas
Resveratrol	Grapes, peanuts, red wine	May reduce the risk of certain cancers such as colorectal, breast, pancreatic	Eat grapes, replace scotch and beer with red wine
Monoterpenes	Citrus fruits (oranges, grapefruits, sweet lemon, lemon)	May activate cancer-causing agents against pancreatic, leukaemia, skin, liver, lung and fore-stomach	Have raw fruits 3 or more times a day
Isoflavones	Soy foods (tofu, soy milk), soybean, legumes, (kidney beans, green moong, black-eyed beans, chickpeas)	Protects against cancers such as lung, breast, gastric, lymphoma	Replace cheese with tofu in sandwiches. Eat lentils as salad, pancakes and gravies with vegetables

Phytochemical in Food	Food Sources	Possible Cancer Benefits	Consumption Ideas
Curcumin and Piperine	Indian spices primarily curcumin and piperine	Keeps cancer at bay and reduces tumour proliferation such as breast and other solid cancers	Add spices to your meals in soups, broths, and curries, in tea, milk, and infused water

Key Takeaways

✓ Cancer treatment requires strict nutritional discipline.

✓ A combination of a healthy diet and nourishing fluids can complement the recovery process.

✓ Eating small portions of food can help deal with nausea and vomiting.

✓ Avoid fatty, greasy, spicy, and strong-smelling foods.

✓ High fibre foods such as whole grains, fresh and cooked vegetables, fresh and dried fruits, and foods containing peels, nuts, and seeds are advised for people complaining of constipation.

✓ Light physical activity like a walk or simple exercise can work wonders for people recovering from cancer.

CHAPTER SIX

Spice Up Your Life
The Ayurveda Way

Sattvic means pure substance. This is the purest eating routine for an intentionally profound and sound life. It sustains the body and keeps it in a peaceful state. As indicated by Ayurveda, this is the best eating routine for physical quality, a great personality, great well-being, and a long lifespan. Furthermore, it quietens and filters the mind, empowering it to work at its highest potential. A sattvic eating regimen subsequently prompts genuine well-being: a cheerful personality responsible for a fit body, with an adjusted stream of vitality between them. A sattvic eating routine is fantastic for those people who want to carry on a calm, tranquil, and reflective life.

Sattvic food includes the eating regimen of numerous sages, yogis, and profound educators. These nourishments should create tranquillity and respectability among men. Articulation of the spirit is subject to the body, and the body is dependent on food. The sattvic eating routine comprises light, calming, effortlessly processed nourishment. Sattvic implies the etheric characteristics and incorporates products of the soil, particularly sun nourishments and ground nourishments. Sattvic nourishments that are sun foods are those that grow one metre or more above the ground. They have a reviving and helping impact on the body's apprehensive and stomach related frameworks. Ground foods are those nourishments that develop on the inside of the ground up to one metre. They draw vitality from the earth and are high in nutrients. Sattvic nourishments incorporate entire grains, fresh organic product, land and ocean vegetables, pure natural product squeezes, nut and seed drain and cheddar, vegetables, nuts, seeds, grew seeds, nectar, and herb teas. As per the eating regimen, the best nourishments are those that are crisp, have a mixture of all the six tastes: sweet, sour, salty, pungent (spicy), bitter, and astringent (driest flavour).

Sattvik foods comprise the following-

Natural products:
Apples, Kiwi, Prunes, Apricots, Tangerines, Bananas, Lychee, Pomegranate, Cantaloupe, Mango, Papaya, Cherries, Melons, Honeydew, Oranges, Grapefruits, Watermelon, Pineapples, Grapes, Peaches, Plums, Guava, Pears, Persimmon

Vegetables:
Artichokes, Eggplant, Lettuce, Beets, Mustard, Greens, Asparagus, Daikon, Onions, Endive, Fennel, Maitake, Parsnips, Bok Choy, Peas, Broccoli, Green Beans, Potatoes, Brussels Sprouts, Kale, Radishes,

Cabbage, Leeks, Lima Beans, Shallots, Carrots, Celery, Spinach, Cauliflower, Sprouts, Corn, Squash, Shitake, Mushrooms, Watercress, Turnips, Yams

Grown Whole Grains:
Amaranth, Barley, Buckwheat, Bulgur, Millet, Quinoa, Rice (Basmati, Brown and Wild Rice)

Oils:
Olive, Mustard, Sesame, Garbanzo, Lentils, Mung

Flavours:
Asafoetida (Hing), Coriander, Basil, Cumin, Nutmeg, Black Pepper, Fennel seed, Parsley, Cardamom, Fenugreek, Turmeric, Cinnamon, Cloves, Ginger

Nut/Seed:
Brazil nuts, Pumpkin seeds, Sunflower seeds, Walnuts, Almonds, Peanuts

It requires time for the impacts of dietary changes to show on the brain. Changing our eating regimen may not affect our brain science overnight, but in a time span of a few months, it can influence it drastically. Envision your food with no flavours. Impossible, is it?

We know that wherever you locate an Indian, you will discover flavours. No big surprise, when food goliaths from over the world come to India, they need to add an Indian contort to their menu. Ideal for the kitchen and therapeutic uses in homes, flavours have a critical part to play in many places. As India is honoured with a changed atmosphere, each one of its states delivers some zest or the other. No big surprise why flavours are utilized so broadly to cook in India. Aside from including spices, flavour, and taste, utilization of flavours in the right way gives endless medical advantages. Let's have a quick review of Indian flavours and their advantages of keeping Ayurveda in perspective.

- **Asafoetida (Hing):** It is utilized for flavouring foods especially snacks and has therapeutic uses. An excellent solution for whooping cough and stomach ache due to flatulence.
- **Bay leaf (Tez Patta):** It is utilized as a part of cooking to add a particular flavour to the food. It likewise has some therapeutic properties. Bay leaf oil has antibacterial and antifungal properties.
- **Cardamom (Elaichi):** It is utilized as a part of a large portion of Indian cooking and making sweet dishes to give a decent flavour and smell. It is additionally used broadly in the pharmaceutical sector. Helps to control awful breath and stomach related confusion.
- **Cinnamon (Dalchini):** It is utilized mostly to season nourishment and as a spice in many Indian dishes. It underpins an improved generation of insulin and decreases blood cholesterol.
- **Clove (Laung):** It is utilized as a cooking ingredient predominantly to season or to get the masalas ready.

Clove oil is helpful for treating toothache and sore gums. It is advantageous for chest torments, fever, stomach related issues, cough, and cold.

- **Coriander (Dhaniya):** Coriander leaves and coriander seeds are utilized as a part of Indian cooking. It additionally has some therapeutic uses. It can be used remotely on throbbing joints and stiffness. It is also useful for a throat infection, hypersensitivities, and absorption issues, to feed the fever and so on.

- **Cumin (Zeera):** Commonly used in cooking and seasoning, it is a decent source of iron and keeps resistant framework sound. Water overflowed with cumin seeds is useful for managing loose bowels.

- **Curry leaves (Curry Patta):** It is utilized as a principal element for flavouring in a few nations. It has numerous therapeutic uses. These leaves can lessen glucose and are a dense source of micronutrients. The dried leaves are widely utilized as a part of home-grown prescriptions.

- **Fenugreek (Methi):** It is primarily utilized as a green vegetable and seeds are used for flavouring in Indian cooking. Fenugreek seed tea or sweet fudge is useful for nursing mothers. It is also used for treating diabetes and bringing down cholesterol.

- **Garlic (Lassan):** It is utilized for cooking as well as for therapeutic purposes. It is helpful for adapting to cold and cough. It has anti-toxin and anti-cancer properties.

- **Ginger (Adrak):** It is utilized for giving a particular flavour to food and has numerous therapeutic uses. It helps the body fight stomach related issues. It is helpful for adapting to cough and cold.

- **Mustard (Rye):** The utilization of mustard oil is widespread in India, yet it is prohibited in some countries. Mustard oil is useful for heart health and helps to nourish and grow fantastic hair. It comprises of omega-3 unsaturated fats. It is an excellent source of iron, zinc, manganese, calcium, and protein.

- **Pepper (Kaali Mirch):** It is widely utilized as a significant part of cooking, particularly to garnish the food. It enables adapting to cold and common flu. It manages muscle agonies and makes digestion robust.

- **Saffron (Zaffran/Kesar):** It is utilized for cooking as well as in luxury food items. It is for the most part used as a part of sweet dishes. It has excellent restorative properties. It adapts to skin maladies. It is a decent solution for cough, cold, and asthma.

- **Turmeric (Haldi):** It is utilized as a part of cooking and is an active ingredient of healthy skin items. It has a wide range of therapeutic uses. It helps to manage skin issues. Turmeric powder can be utilized for mending cuts and wounds. It additionally makes adapting to diabetes less demanding. Curcumin in turmeric has anti-cancer and anti-inflammatory properties.

Cleaning the Air around Ayurveda

Ayurveda has never been so commercially exploited as in the present times. Almost every FMCG brand has come up with Ayurveda-based products that boast of miraculous health benefits. While brands have restricted Ayurveda to a collection of some complicated and unspellable natural herbs, I'll try to introduce Ayurveda to you in its unadulterated form.

World-renowned Ayurvedic physician Vasant Lad writes in his book, *The Complete Book of Ayurvedic Home Remedies*, "As a science of self-healing, Ayurveda encompasses diet and nutrition, lifestyle exercise, rest and relaxation, meditation, breathing exercises, and medicinal herbs, along with cleansing and rejuvenation programs for healing body, mind, and spirit."

Tridoshas—The Fundamental Principles of Ayurveda

Ayurveda dwells on three dynamic principles referred to as tridoshas—vata, pitta, and kapha, which govern one's mind, body, and consciousness. Ayurveda aims to achieve a state of health where there is a harmony between these doshas or fundamental energies.

Ayurveda, a Sanskrit word meaning the 'science of life and longevity', sees each individual as a constitution or prakruti, constituted of five universal energies—ether, air, fire, water, and earth. These five elements combine to govern and regulate tridoshas within an individual or prakruti.

Ether and air combine to constitute vata dosha, the fire and water elements together attribute to pitta dosha, and earth and water elements in combination regulate kapha dosha.

Let's dig deeper into the tridoshas to understand how they influence prakruti or simply an individual's body functions. As we discussed earlier, tridoshas together are responsible for regulating all biological, physiopathological, and psychological functions of one's mind, body, and consciousness. They also stimulate an individual's natural urges while governing his or her eating preferences. In simple words, the individual choices like the taste, temperatures, and likes and dislikes in eating are all governed by tridoshas. Whatever happens in our body including production and maintenance of body tissues, digestion, secretion and excretion, etc., all happens at the state of tridosha. To the surprise of many, our emotions like anger, fear, and greed, etc., are at the mercy of these three.

Overall, all's well inside our body until these three components are in harmony. And, once they are out of balance, the development of diseases begins.

The following depicts the position of tridoshas in our body:

The Seats of Vata, Pitta, Kapha

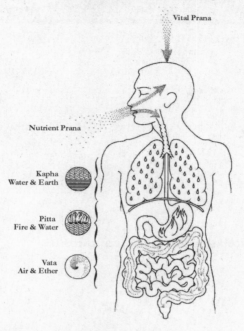

(Source: *Ayurveda: The Science of Self Healing:*
A Practical Guide by Vasant Lad)

Let's have a look at the following table to understand the function of each dosha:

Vatta (Air+Space)	Pitta (Fire+Water)	Kapha (Water+Earth)
Movement	Body Heat	Stability
Breathing	Temperature	Energy
Natural Urges	Digestion	Lubrication

Vatta (Air+Space)	Pitta (Fire+Water)	Kapha (Water+Earth)
Transformation of Tissues	Perception	Unctuousness
Motor Functions	Understanding	Forgiveness
Sensory Functions	Hunger	Greed
Ungroundedness	Thirst	Attachment
Secretions	Intelligence	Accumulation
Excretions	Anger	Holding
Fear	Hate	Possessiveness
Emptiness	Jealousy	
Anxiety		

Interrelationship between tridoshas

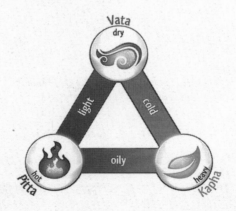

The diagram shows oiliness as the common link between pitta and kapha. Pitta and vata share light as the common link while vata and kapha have cold in common.

In a nutshell, Ayurveda aims to heal a constitution or prakruti by achieving a balance in the internal forces or doshas through healthy changes in diet and eating habits so that the body can cope with the dynamics of the external environment.

Famous Ayurvedic Physician, Vasant Lad, writes in his book *Ayurveda: The Science of Self Healing: A Practical Guide:*

"Together, the tridosha governs all metabolic activities: anabolism (kapha), catabolism (vata), and metabolism (pitta). When vata is out of balance, the metabolism will be disturbed, resulting in excess catabolism, which is the breakdown or deterioration process in the body. When anabolism is greater than catabolism, there is an increased rate of growth and repair of the organs and tissues. Excess pitta disturbs metabolism, excess kapha increases the rate of anabolism and excess vata creates emaciation (catabolism)."

How to determine your constitution (prakruti)

- Indications of a vata constitution (to be elaborated)
- Indications of pitta constitution (to be elaborated)
- Indications of kapha constitution (to be elaborated)

Personal Traits as per Tridoshas

Aspect of the Constitution	Vata	Pitta	Kapha
Frame	Thin	Moderate	Thick
Body Weight	Low	Moderate	Overweight

Aspect of the Constitution	Vata	Pitta	Kapha
Skin	Dry, Rough, Cool, Brown, Black	Soft, Oily, Warm, Fair, Red, Yellowish	Thick, Oily, Cool, Pale, White
Hair	Black, Dry	Soft, Oily, Yellow, Early Grey, Red	Thick, oily, wavy, Dark or Light
Teeth	Protruded, Big and Crooked, Gums Emaciated	Moderate in Size, Soft Gums, Yellowish	Strong White
Eyes	Small, Dull, Dry, Brown Black	Sharp, Penetrating Green, Grey, Yellow	Big, Attractive, Blue, Thick Eyelashes
Appetite	Variable, Scanty	Good, Excessive, Unbearable	Slow but steady
Taste	Sweet, Sour, Saline	Sweet, Bitter, Astringent	Pungent, Bitter, Astringent
Thirst	Variable	Excessive	Scanty
Elimination	Dry, Hard Constipated	Soft, Oily, Loose	Thick, Oily, Heavy, Slow
Physical Activity	Very Active	Moderate	Lethargic

Aspect of the Constitution	Vata	Pitta	Kapha
Mind	Restless Active	Aggressive, Intelligent	Calm, Slow
Emotional Temperament	Fearful, Insecure, Unpredictable	Aggressive, Irritable, Jealous	Calm, Greedy, Attached
Faith	Changeable	Fanatic	Steady
Memory	Recent Memory: Good Remote Memory: Poor	Sharp	Slow but Prolonged
Dreams	Fearful, Flying, Jumping, Running	Fiery, Anger, Violence, War	Watery, River, Ocean, Lake, Swimming, Romantic
Sleep	Scanty, Interrupted	Little but Sound	Heavy, Prolonged
Speech	Fast	Sharp and Cutting	Slow, Monotonous
Financial Status	Poor, Spends money quickly on trifles	Moderate, Spends on luxuries	Rich, Moneysaver, Spends on food
Pulse	Thready, Feeble moves like a snake	Moderate, Jumping like a frog	Broad, Slow, Moves like a swan

Ayurveda and Diet

Ayurveda believes in one's power to heal oneself. Therefore, this ancient science of healing guides all individuals to take care of their health by understanding their body's constitution and its requirements. Ayurveda recommends maintaining a healthy diet supplemented by a stable healthy lifestyle to enjoy optimum health and wellness. In addition, it also advises the traditional relaxation techniques including yoga and breathing exercises as well as the 'spiritual practices' in order to live a harmonious and happy life.

Talking about the food, Ayurveda prescribes a diet compatible with your constitution or prakruti. According to Ayurveda, there are six rasas or tastes of food—sweet, salty, pungent, sour, bitter, and astringent. In addition, it categorizes food as heat- or cold-producing, heavy or light, liquid or solid, and oily or dry. Ayurveda also advises to consider the season while choosing your foods.

The following table offers recommended foods suitable for different constitution types:

Types of Constitutions

Types of Foods	Vata		Pitta		Kapha	
	Aggravates Dosha	Balances Dosha	Aggravates Dosha	Balances Dosha	Aggravates Dosha	Balances Dosha
Fruits	Dried fruits Apples Cranberries Pears Persimmon Pomegranate Watermelon	Sweet fruits Apricots Avocados Bananas Berries Cherries Coconut Figs (fresh) Grapefruit Grapes Lemons Mango Melons (sweet) Oranges Papaya Peaches Pineapples Plums	Sour fruits Apricots Berries Bananas Cherries Cranberries Grapefruit Grapes (green) Lemons Oranges (sour) Papaya Peaches Pineapples (sour) Plums (sour)	Sweet Fruits Apples Avocados Coconut Figs Grapes (dark) Mango Melons Oranges (sweet) Pears Pineapples (sweet) Plums (sweet) Pomegranate Prunes Raisins	Sweet & sour fruits Avocado Bananas Coconut Figs (fresh) Grapefruit Grapes Lemons Melons Oranges Papaya Pineapples Plums	Apples Apricots Berries Cherries Cranberries Figs (dry) Mango Peaches Pears Pomegranate Prunes Raisins

Types of Foods	Vata		Pitta		Kapha	
	Aggravates Dosha	Balances Dosha	Aggravates Dosha	Balances Dosha	Aggravates Dosha	Balances Dosha
Vegetables	Raw vegetables Broccoli Brussels sprouts Cabbage Cauliflower Celery Eggplant Mushrooms Onions (raw) Peas Peppers Potatoes (white) Tomatoes	Cooked vegetables Asparagus Beets Carrots Cucumber Garlic Green beans Okra (cooked) Onion (cooked) Potato (sweet) Radishes Zucchini	Pungent vegetables Beets Carrots Eggplant Garlic Onions Peppers (hot) Radishes Spinach Tomatoes	Sweet & bitter vegetables Asparagus Broccoli Brussels sprouts Cabbage Cauliflower Celery Cucumber Green beans Leafy greens Lettuce Mushrooms Okra Peas Parsley Peppers (green) Potatoes Sprouts Zucchini	Sweet & juicy vegetables Cucumber Potatoes (sweet) Tomatoes Zucchini	Pungent & bitter vegetables Asparagus Beets Broccoli Brussels sprouts Cabbage Carrots Cauliflower Celery Eggplant Garlic Leafy greens Lettuce Mushrooms Okra Onions Parsley Peas Peppers Potatoes (white) Radishes Spinach Sprouts

Types of Foods	Vata Aggravates Dosha	Vata Balances Dosha	Pitta Aggravates Dosha	Pitta Balances Dosha	Kapha Aggravates Dosha	Kapha Balances Dosha
Grains	Barley Buckwheat Corn Millet Oats (dry) Rye	Oats (cooked) Rice Wheat	Buckwheat Corn Millet Oats (dry) Rice (brown) Rye	Barley Oats (cooked) Rice (basmati) Rice (white) Wheat	Oats (cooked) Rice (brown) Rice (white) Wheat	Barley Corn Millet Oats (dry) Rice (basmati small amount) Rye
Legumes	No legumes except moong beans and black and red lentils		All legumes are okay except lentils		All legumes are good except kidney beans, soybeans, black lentils, and mung beans	
Nuts	All nuts are okay in small quantities		No nuts except coconut		No nuts at all	
Seeds	All seeds are okay but in moderation		No seeds except sunflower and pumpkin		No seeds except sunflower and pumpkin	
Sweeteners	All sweeteners are okay except white sugar		All sweets are okay except molasses and honey		No sweeteners except raw honey	
Condiments	All spices are good		No spices except cinnamon, coriander, fennel, cardamom, turmeric and black pepper in a small amount		All spices are good except salt	

Types of Foods	Vata		Pitta		Kapha	
	Aggravates Dosha	Balances Dosha	Aggravates Dosha	Balances Dosha	Aggravates Dosha	Balances Dosha
Dairy		All dairy products are okay in moderation	NO Buttermilk Cheese Sour cream Yoghurt	YES Butter (unsalted) Cottage cheese Ghee Milk	No dairy except ghee and goatmilk	
Oils		All oils are good	NO Almond Corn Safflower Sesame	YES Coconut Olive Sunflower Soy	No oils except almond, corn, or sunflower in small amounts	

Food interactions in Ayurveda

Ayurveda is very particular about food interactions (reactions that take place after one consumes two or more foods that are non-compatible to each other) which are associated with many disorders.

For example, Ayurveda principles prohibit the consumption of fish and milk together as it may cause problems including constipation, blood-borne diseases, obstruction of channels of circulation, vitiation of blood, and even death. Similarly, intake of meat of aquatic, domestic, and marshy animals in combination with food products like sugar candy, milk, honey, sesame seeds, radish, and lotus stalk, etc., is believed to cause many problems such as blindness, trembling, deafness, dumbness, loss of intelligence, and even death.

Consuming hot food after taking pork, eating sour foods with milk, intake of honey and ghee in equal quantity and intake of cold foods after taking ghee is associated with various health problems such as fainting, intoxication, skin diseases, blindness, sterility, oedema, rhinitis, fever and even death. Similarly, there are many proposed food interactions that Ayurveda refers to as dangerous and suggests to avoid them.

Food combinations to Reduce or Avoid

The accompanying rundown features different nourishments and offers recommendations for more proper blends. It is intended to be a useful guide, not a thorough summary. You might know about different mixes that don't work for your body. Respect those senses. Since this asset is intended to enable you to decide ideal combinations initially, there is some redundancy. Indeed, a portion of these staples blends in numerous family units. Pizza and various other darling Italian dishes consolidate nightshades with cheddar.

Furthermore, who among us hasn't appreciated beans with cheddar at some point or other? At that point, there are the foods grown from the ground forbidden. We should make sure that what we eat is soothing our body and not ruining it.

	Incompatible Foods:	Supportive Combinations:
Beans	Fruit, milk, cheese, yoghurt, eggs, meat, fish	Grains, vegetables, other beans, nuts, seeds
Dairy	Depends on the type of dairy; see individual categories below	
Butter & Ghee	Butter may not combine with other foods as universally as ghee	Grains, vegetables, beans, nuts, seeds, meat, fish, eggs, cooked fruit
Cheese	Fruit, beans, eggs, milk, yoghurt, hot drinks	Grains, vegetables

	Incompatible Foods:	Supportive Combinations:
Milk	Any other food (especially bananas, cherries, melons, sour fruits, yeasted breads, eggs, yoghurt, meat, fish, khichdi, starches)	Milk is best enjoyed alone . . . Exceptions: rice pudding, oatmeal, dates, almonds
Yoghurt	Fruit, beans, milk, cheese, eggs, meat, fish, nightshades, hot drinks	Vegetables, grains
Eggs	Milk, cheese, yoghurt, fruit (especially melons), beans, kitchari, potatoes, meat, fish	Grains, non-starchy vegetables
Fruits	Any other food (aside from other fruit) *Exceptions: dates with milk, some cooked combinations	Other fruits with similar qualities (citrus together, apples with pears, a berry medley, etc.)
Lemons	Cucumbers, tomatoes, milk, yoghurt Note: lime can be substituted for use with cucumbers and tomatoes	Usually okay with other foods, if used in small amounts as a garnish or flavouring

	Incompatible Foods:	Supportive Combinations:
Melons	Everything (especially dairy, eggs, fried food, grains, starches) *More than most fruit, melons should be eaten alone or not at all	Other melons (in a pinch) . . . But it's better to have each type of melon on its own
Grains	Fruit	Beans, vegetables, other grains, eggs, meat, fish, nuts, seeds, cheese, yoghurt
Vegetables	Fruit, milk	Grains, beans, other vegetables, cheese, yoghurt, meat, fish, nuts, seeds, eggs
Nightshades	Fruit (especially melon), cucumber, milk, cheese, yoghurt. Note: nightshades include peppers, eggplant, potatoes, and tomatoes	Other vegetables, grains, beans, meat, fish, nuts, seeds

In a Nutshell

How many of us knew that honey becomes harmful when cooked? Cooked or warmed nectar takes longer to process, and its atoms wind up stuck to mucous layer and bolt narrow channels, delivering poison.

There are so many things that we eat daily in our day-to-day activities, and we don't even realize the benefits of it and the purity it provides us.

Ayurveda has been a part of our lives without us even knowing about it; it is there in the food we eat and the habits we possess and has been ever since bringing a significant improvement in our lives.

To end with, there is a regular Ayurveda activity that you should indulge in, and that is a self-massage: Massaging at least one of the vitality channels with fragrant oil surges the psyche and body with recuperating vitality.

Ayurveda is a study that warms up our life, and if followed with absolute dedication, it can completely change the way we live and make our lives healthier, happier, and nourished.

CHAPTER SEVEN

Ready to Diet: Unpleasant Surprises of Packaged Food

Chetan is from Chitoor, a small town fifty kilometres from Vijaywada. He has come to New Delhi to pursue his career in the corporate industry. He works with Wipro technologies in New Delhi as a customer care professional. His office timings are from 6 pm to 3 am.

Chetan decides to stay in a rented apartment but decides to cook his own food. But contrary to his desires, due to his office timings, Chetan is forced to eat packaged food all the way from Tetra Pak milk to juices to biscuits to all the junk food available. In the mornings he drinks Tetra Pak milk and goes to sleep. Post that he wakes up at 2 pm, dizzy, wanting to eat something healthy for lunch, but is forced to eat the ready-to-cook MTR parantha and Dal makhani. The cost of the food is Rs 120 only for both the items and Chetan eats the meal. By 5 pm he has to leave for office.

The dinner served in the office is not of high quality as there are only fried items like samosa available, so Chetan is forced to eat packaged food and is now accustomed to it. The cycle keeps on repeating and Chetan develops a taste for packaged food. What he does not realize is that his health is deteriorating day by day. Not only has he gained weight and feels low on energy but has also got into the habit of eating packaged food where the nutrition is inadequate to suffice his needs. This excess or daily consumption of packaged food is wreaking havoc with his health and can also lead to illness in the long run.

Origin of Packaged Food

There was a time when men used to simply consume what they found edible in their immediate surroundings. And then we learnt the art of cooking. We started preparing fresh food and consuming it before it could lose its warmth and taste. But, things started to change as men learnt the art and science of food packaging.

Origin

The earliest account of packaging is known to be present in the pre-historic period when he started to live in caves. It was the first time he felt the need for food storage. Initially, the early man used leaves, shells, and gourds to meet his storage needs. It was before the time he learnt to weave baskets using wood, grasses, and bamboo as the raw material. Historians report the first manufacturing of glass and pottery in 7000 BC. Interestingly, the raw materials (including silica, limestone, soda, and sand) for making storage containers are the same today as it was thousands of years ago.

Early Development in Packaging

In the late eighteenth century when the Industrial Revolution in Europe and the US took the world by storm, new materials and manufacturing processes evolved. Some of these materials like cans, that were not initially intended for storage, served as storage containers—for their ability to block moisture and retain the flavour of the food item. Nicolas Appert, a French innovator, is credited with the development of airtight containers for food storage. His discovery of airtight metal cans solved French Emperor Napolean Bonaparte's problem to preserve food for his army. Appert's metal cans used for storing food could be heated conveniently, thereby improving the shelf life of the food stored.

Although plastic materials including vinyl chloride, styrene, and cellulose nitrate had been developed by 1800s, they did not find their application in food storage until the twentieth century. The first use of plastic material for food packaging was seen in World War II when it served the purpose at a commercial scale. Before that, a major development in the food packaging industry was recorded in 1892 when William Painter, the founder of today's Crown Holdings, Inc., patented the crown cork. The innovation brought a boom in the beverage industry. A metal cap fitted with a layer of rubber cork, crown cork provided an airtight means to cap the beverage-filled bottles. Over time, plastics and other synthetic materials replaced the cork, providing a tighter and reliable seal, resisting the ingress of oxygen in the bottle and protecting the product from deterioration.

In addition to beverages, biscuits were among the first ones in packaged foods. National Biscuit Co., formed by the merger of different baking companies, became the first company to start selling packaged biscuits in the 1890s. The company broke the tradition of selling loose biscuits stored in large barrels and introduced small SKUs of lighter and flakier biscuits, packaged in moisture-proof packages.

World War II and Commercialization of Packaged Food

Before World War II, packaged food was largely limited to biscuits and beverages. It was in WWII when the concept of canned food gained prominence. It was the time when our day-to-day food started coming in cans with a longer shelf life. Canned food that kick-started a revolution in the packaged food industry was originally developed during this time for American soldiers so that the additional efforts required to cook food in the warzone could be saved.

Packaged food industry flourished post-WWII

The conclusion of WWII left the manufacturers with huge stores of canned food, which they started selling in supermarkets. To ensure that they don't incur losses on surplus stock, they began an aggressive marketing campaign to sell canned and other packaged foods to middle-class civilian consumers. And in no time, packaged food penetrated the busy lifestyles of Americans and became an inexpensive and instant alternative to feed oneself.

While the WWII ended in 1945, the success story of packaged food as a prospering industry began.

Soon, processed foods became household food instead of just war food. Manufacturers had now started producing these foods ranging from cured meats, to powdered cheeses, to instant drinks, for the civilian market.

The new leaders of the packaged food industry now wanted to run viable and profitable businesses. For which they started offering highly standardized products at affordable costs. The second half of the twentieth century saw a big leap in this market. Women had come out of their kitchens and were contributing to the family's income by taking jobs outside. However, it had left them with very limited time to take care of their children and households. Entrepreneurs saw it as a great business opportunity and started working to offer fast and tasty snacks that could be prepared and consumed in quick time. As the standard of living improved, women preferred eating at restaurants than cooking at home.

Soon, feminist movements aimed at liberating women from the cumbersome and time-consuming process of cooking started doing rounds all over America. As a result, the ready-made food became the new norm and home-cooked food took a backseat, which gave birth to a new term called 'fast-food' meaning that food can be cooked and served in quick time. In no time, the country was full of restaurants that served fast-food.

Now that both men and women were working they had more money to spend on luxuries and eating out was one among them. Seeing the growing demand, the restaurants started thinking of new ideas to have an edge over their competitors. And, at the same time, America had started receiving immigrants, which prompted the restaurants to start serving different types of cuisines including British, Italian, Japanese, Chinese, and Mexican.

As fast-food became popular, voices complaining of adverse effects of fast-food also started getting louder. Soon, there were studies that showed that fast-food restaurants were serving food containing high levels of trans fats, which could lead to various health problems including diabetes, obesity, and cardiovascular problems. Trends showed a drastic increase in the number of overweight people in the United States. The incidence of obese population witnessed a whopping increase, from only 9% in the 1950s to 30.5% in 2000, thanks to high-calorie intake. It is estimated men and women consumed around 2200 and 1500 calories respectively during that time.

Though fast-food continued to enjoy the limelight, some serious studies about the harmful effects of fast-food made people take notice of their health, especially those who had started to experience lifestyle-related problems. As a result, they started to look for healthy food options. Soon, food products boasting of healthy packaged foods flooded the market befooling the consumers once again.

Post WWII, the surplus stock of the canned or the processed food made its way to the restaurants and grocery stores in towns and cities. Seeing the growing demand for it, the manufacturers gave their all to capitalize on this newly developed business opportunity. McDonald's was among the first movers to jump onto the bandwagon with its series of fast-food restaurants that offered reasonable products at affordable prices. While these foods were growing in popularity, studies holding these foods responsible for causing health problems such as diabetes, cardiovascular problems, cancers, obesity, and musculoskeletal disorders were also doing rounds.

While researchers continued to criticize processed foods, manufacturers came up with marketing campaigns that washed away their logic and a product portfolio that pleased their palates to the extent that they couldn't think beyond the taste. Let's understand how these new-age food manufacturers made consumers the slaves of taste.

The Craft of Taste Engineering

Michael Moss, in his Pulitzer Prize-winning book *Salt Sugar Fat: How the Food Giants Hooked Us*, writes about these traders of taste, which served unhealthy food to consumers in the name of taste. He explained how smart food technicians were responsible for addiction to junk foods, which children started to develop at a very young age. He refers to Julie Mennella's (a biopsychologist) extensive researcher on children's love for sugar. She discovered that food technicians while zeroing in on the perfect formulas for their products, ranging from carbonated beverages to potato chips, privately refer to a unique parameter called 'bliss point'.

The bliss point refers to the precise quantity of sweetness (no more, no less) that makes these food products enjoyable and pleasant to the taste buds.

The foods developed through this formula of bliss point made consumers slave to the taste. As a result, they started making their food choices based on how the foods feel in their mouths and not on the basis of their nutritious value.

Let me give you the scientific reason for these preferences. Every time we find something 'tasty' in our mouths, our brain discharges the signal of pleasure as a reward for choosing that food. This phenomenon is similar to developing an addiction to intoxicating substances. And that's why we have that strong craving for foods we know will be flavourful.

The Bitter Taste of Salt

In the 1980s when cases of high blood pressure skyrocketed, the researchers were after the culprit. Doctors and scientists held several meetings to catch the cause of this sudden increase in the incidence of this 'silent killer'. While they could not find the precise cause, they ended up zeroing in on certain factors that may lead to the epidemic called high blood pressure. The key factors identified were obesity, diabetes, and smoking. Another factor that was a surprise inclusion was salt. It may not be a big surprise to people in today's time but at that time people could not believe the pinch of salt they added to their food could give them a heart attack.

Actually, salt per se is not the problem. The problem lies in one of the chemicals present in the salt—sodium. While a little quantity of sodium is a requisite for our body, too much of it can be harmful. And, the fact that Americans were consuming too much salt, their bodies were unable to deal with the extra sodium they were getting, which, in turn, was contributing to high blood pressure, the researchers revealed.

Initially, experts blamed the saltshakers that graced all dining tables of America. And soon, every health professional was after those poor saltshakers without ensuring if sodium present in the table salt was the actual culprit. However, soon researchers realized that table salt alone could not wreak such havoc. And, they once again engaged in their studies to trace the source of sodium damaging the hearts of people.

Surprisingly, the so-called weight-loss diets or the low-fat, low-sugar versions for diabetes management foods were delivering salt in high doses, revealed researchers.

In 1991, a new study published in the *Journal of the American College of Nutrition* cleared the air around the reason of increased salt intake. The researchers had finally nailed the real culprit—packaged food. It was found that natural sodium present in their food plus the salt sprinkled from the saltshaker only contributed to a fifth of the salt they consumed in total. The researchers revealed that over three-quarters of the salt they consumed in the week came from processed foods including canned spaghetti and meatballs, heat-and-serve meals, tomato sauces, salad dressings, pizzas, and soups. Surprisingly, the so-called weight-loss diets or the low-fat, low-sugar versions for diabetes management foods were delivering salt in high doses.

Unfortunately, salt is not the only way processed food manufacturers deliver sodium into our body. Sodium is also used as a food additive into the processed food for purposes other than providing salty taste. A number of sodium-based compounds make their way into the processed food to bind ingredients, delay the bacterial activity and to blend mixtures that otherwise remain unglued. It may make your ready-made food feel fresh, look ravishing, and taste amazing but ultimately it is going to trouble your heart. In the game of taste, your taste buds may win but health will lose.

What's bad in this scenario is that manufacturers are completely ignorant of what their products are doing to people's health. All they are bothered about is their profits and serving their toxic food to the consumers in the name of taste.

Did Sugar Industry Play Foul In 1960s?

A study published in early 2018 made some startling revelations on how the sugar industry in the 1960s made 'fat' the main culprit. The study claims the sugar manufacturers in that time paid the scientists to play down the role of sugar in causing heart-related ailments while shifting the whole blame on saturated fats.

While a majority of studies at that time were holding fats guilty of the growing waistline and weakened hearts of the Americans, the contribution of sugar remained hidden or miserly reported. For decades, people continued to believe that reducing their fat intake is the best way to stay healthy and fit. As a result, people shifted to a low-fat, high-sugar diet, which now experts believe was among the major reasons to fuel obesity. It is estimated that consumption of soft drinks grew five times between 1950 and 2000. Soft drinks and fruit drinks contain around 50% of added sugars like glucose and fructose.

However, things started to change after some researchers came up with unbiased studies bringing to light the harmful effects of sugar too. Studies have linked the consumption of sugar-sweetened beverages to the increased risk of metabolic syndrome, cardiovascular disease, and obesity. High sugar intake is also known to cause non-alcoholic fatty liver disease and increased triglycerides levels. Another study suggested that intake of sugar-sweetened beverages, particularly soda, was associated with increased weight gain.

WHO Changes the Guidelines

Seeing the health hazards of the excess sugar in the packaged food, even the World Health Organization (WHO) had to change its guidelines on the amount of sugar intake in our diet. According to the new guidelines issued in 2015, the WHO recommends adults and children to not consume free sugars more than 10% of their total energy consumption. A further cut down to 25 grams (6 teaspoons) or 5% of the total energy consumption is associated with more benefits. Free sugars, according to the WHO, comprise disaccharides (including table sugar or sucrose) and monosaccharides (like fructose and glucose) added to foods and beverages, and sugars naturally present in fruit juices, honey, syrups, and fruit juice concentrates.

In Geneva, on March 4, 2015, the WHO issued a new guideline to reduce the daily intake of free sugars for adults and children. "We have solid evidence that keeping intake of free sugars to less than 10% of total energy intake reduces the risk of overweight, obesity, and tooth decay. Making policy changes to support this will be key if countries are to live up to their commitments to reduce the burden of noncommunicable diseases," explained Dr Francesco Branca, Director of WHO's Department of Nutrition for Health and Development.

It is important to note that sugars naturally present in milk and the sugars in vegetables and fresh fruits do not fall under WHO guidelines, as there is no known association between these sugars and any possible adverse effects.

WHO is very particular about sugars 'hidden' in processed foods. Generally, people are ignorant of this type of sugar as they mostly relate sugar to sweets or sweetened products. For instance, free sugars present in 1 tablespoon of ketchup amount to around 1 teaspoon, roughly 4 grams.

Similarly, one can of sugar-sweetened soda delivers around 10 teaspoons or 40 grams free sugars.

Daily dietary habits of a typical corporate guy

A normal corporate guy is always short of time. And the thing that is most affected is his diet. Having left with very little time to eat home-cooked food, he dwells on mostly packaged and convenient foods, accompanied by sweet carbonated beverages.

Let's see how the daily food menu of a busy working professional looks like:

Breakfast (7:30 am)
- Breakfast cereals, muesli oats
- Whole grain toast
- Factory butter/spread
- Packed juice

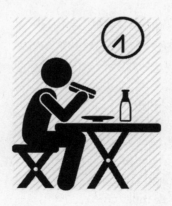

Morning Snacks (11:00 am)
- Starbucks coffee with creams
- Whole-wheat muffin

Lunch (1:30 pm)
- Regular lunch (Roti, rice, vegetable, etc.)
- Pizzas, burger and outside food (at least once or twice a week)
- Evening snacks
- Fruits/Sprout/Nuts
- Ready-made soups (cuppa soup)
- Tea/coffee

Dinner (7:30 pm)
- Instant noodles
- Ready-to-eat sandwich
- Ready-to-eat biryani/lentil/paneer
- Pre-cooked chapattis (frozen)
- Tetra Pak milk/curd

Key observations

Nearly 40% of the diet a normal corporate person consumes every day comes from the packaged industry. Experts suggest a number of harmful effects of different ingredients present in the packaged food:

Salt: The very high salt levels of salt present in the foods may adversely affect your heart.

Refined flour: Most of the packaged foods contain a high amount of refined flour which may appear pleasant to taste buds but it is associated with increased risk of obesity and risk of cardiovascular diseases.

Added preservatives and taste enhancers: Preservatives and synthetic chemicals present in pre-cooked foods may cause chronic conditions like diabetes, cancer, obesity, and inflammatory and neurological disorders.

Taste enhancing substances (rewarding taste): makes one eat larger portion sizes, thereby magnifying the related risk. Some of the common taste enhancers include monosodium glutamate (MSG), NaCl, and sweeteners that are used to add additional taste or improve palatability to the packaged foods. In addition, sodium benzoate is also used in the production of canned soda while potassium nitrate is used as a colour fixative and antimicrobial agent that increases the shelf life of the foods. Studies suggest that these taste enhancers and additives can adversely affect the biological system of humans.

High sugar: The concept of sugar, for many, is limited to sucrose, the white crystals used for sweetening your cup of tea, coffee, and other dishes. But, sucrose is only the one type of sugar consumed by people. You will be surprised to know that there are around 56 names that can be used for this sweet product. While sucrose is deliberately added to food products, there is added sugar hidden in many products that people are ignorant of while consuming those products. In the United States, nearly 80% of grocery items contain added sugar.

A study published in the journal *PLoS One* in 2007 suggested that intense sugar has higher addictive potential than cocaine. Overconsumption of sugar-dense foods or beverages is initially motivated by the pleasure of sweet taste and is often compared to drug addiction, according to the study.

Here is a list of some foods that contain more sugar than you would have expected:

Product	Sugar Content per 100 gms
Instant Sweetened Lemon Tea	95.3 gms
Milk Chocolate	52.8 gms
Jam	52.3 gms
Chocolate Spread	50 gms
Chocolate Digestive Biscuit	29.2 gms
Tomato Ketchup	23.7 gms
Ice Cream (vanilla)	21 gms
Brown Sauce	19 gms

Product	Sugar Content per 100 gms
Sweet & Sour Sauce	19 gms
Salad Cream	17.5 gms
Fruit Yoghurt	13 gms
Cranberry Juice	11.6 gms
Common Carbonated Beverages	10.6 gms
Cornflakes	8 gms

In addition to the above listed foods, some foods with the 'healthy' tag have high sugar content. Cereals from a popular brand were found to contain 56% of sugar. Similarly, so-called healthy and nutritious Fruit and Nut muesli contains 31% sugar while instant chocolate comprises 60% of sugar. Although fruits and vegetable also contain sugar, they are rich in dietary fibre that helps slow down glucose absorption, thereby mitigating its health risk. Packaged foods like soft drinks, on the contrary, have no nutritious value and are just the sources of sugar.

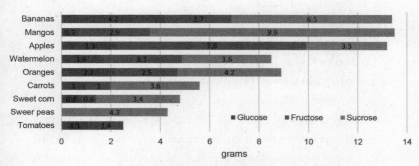

Amount of sugar in fruits (per 100 gms)

Hazards of Added Sugar

According to a research by the University of California-San Francisco, high intake of sugar is associated with increased risk of type 2 diabetes. High doses of sugar increase the body's resistance to insulin produced by the pancreas. The continued consumption of sugar over time may affect the pancreas' ability to generate a sufficient amount of insulin. That in turn, will decrease the level of glucose in the blood, thereby leading to type 2 diabetes.

The second known problem associated with excessive sugar intake is obesity. It occurs when one's weight exceeds 35% of normal body mass, which is an outcome of the conversion of sugar into fat. First dextrose converts to fatty acids, then to triglycerides, and finally stored in a body as adipose tissue. A study appeared in the Journal of the American Medical Association (AMA) revealed that people who receive 25% or more calories from added sugar have over three times higher risk of developing a heart attack, heart disease, or stroke over people who receive less than 5% of calories from sugars. Moreover, AMA suggests an association between a high fructose diet and increased levels of blood pressure. High sugar intake and the resultant high fat deposits increases one's risk of non-alcoholic fatty liver disease, elevated cholesterol levels, high blood pressure, accelerated ageing, digestive disorders, weakened immune system, hyperactivity in children, asthma, migraines, blood clots, osteoporosis, food allergies, kidney damage, mineral deficiencies, and depression.

What's the Problem with Sugar?

1. **Sugar is Linked to Heart Disease**
    High sugar can cause obesity, inflammation, and more issues that can lead to deadly diseases over time. It's also all too easy to consume too much sugar. Just a single can of soda exceeds the recommended daily sugar limit, putting people at risk.

2. **Sugar Causes Weight Gain**
    Today, sugar, not fat, is thought to be the major cause of obesity around the world.

    When you consume simple sugars like fructose, you actually start to feel hungry and want to eat more, rather than feeling satiated. Fructose can even affect the hormones that tell your body when to stop eating, so your body can't properly regulate hunger anymore.

    This is worst in sugary drinks, since they don't address your hunger, but they add to your daily sugar consumption. People are more likely to eat more than they need when they're also consuming a lot of sugar in their beverages.

3. **Sugar Leads to Diabetes**
    Sugar has also been linked to higher rates of diabetes.

    Since obesity is the biggest diabetes risk factors, and sugar has been shown to cause obesity, reducing sugar consumption can also reduce the rates of diabetes. Consuming a lot of sugar leads to insulin resistance, causing high blood sugar levels that increase the risk of diabetes.

4. **Sugar is Linked to Depression**

Sugar intake has also been linked to higher rates of depression. Depression makes it hard for people to get motivated to work out and make lifestyle changes, creating a negative loop of mental and physical illness.

Research has shown that people who eat a lot of sugar are more likely to become depressed. However, a healthy diet can counteract this effect by boosting your mood.

5. **Sugar Has Been Linked to Acne**

A diet high in refined carbs, including sugary foods and drinks, has been associated with a higher risk of developing acne. Foods with a high glycaemic index, such as processed sweets, raise your blood sugar more rapidly than foods with a lower glycaemic index. Sugary foods quickly spike blood sugar and insulin levels, causing increased androgen secretion, oil production, and inflammation, all of which play a role in acne development.

6. **Sugar May Increase Your Risk of Cancer**

Eating excessive amounts of sugar may increase your risk of developing certain cancers. First, a diet rich in sugary foods and beverages can lead to obesity, which significantly raises your risk of cancer. Furthermore, diets high in sugar increase inflammation in your body and may cause insulin resistance, both of which increase cancer risk.

7. **Sugar May Accelerate the Skin Ageing Process**
Wrinkles are a natural sign of ageing. They appear eventually, regardless of your health. However, poor food choices can worsen wrinkles and speed the skin ageing process. Advanced glycation end products are compounds formed by reactions between sugar and protein in your body. They are suspected to play a key role in skin ageing. Consuming a diet high in refined carbs and sugar leads to the production of AGEs, which may cause your skin to age prematurely. AGEs damage collagen and elastin, which are proteins that help the skin stretch and keep its youthful appearance. When collagen and elastin become damaged, the skin loses its firmness and begins to sag.

8. **Sugar Can Lead to Fatty Liver**
A high intake of fructose has been consistently linked to an increased risk of fatty liver. Unlike glucose and other types of sugar, which are taken up by many cells throughout the body, fructose is almost exclusively broken down by the liver. In the liver, fructose is converted into energy or stored as glycogen.

However, the liver can only store so much glycogen before excess amounts are turned into fat. Large amounts of added sugar in the form of fructose overload your liver, leading to non-alcoholic fatty liver disease (NAFLD), a condition characterized by an excessive fat build-up in the liver.

Sugar Industry Scandal: Funding Science To Blame Fat

- Sugar research foundation, as early as 1950, sponsors the first CHD research project
- By 1965 the project is published in leading public journals. It singles out fat and cholesterol as the cause of dietary CHD and downplays evidence that sucrose consumption was a bigger risk factor
- WHO and AHA adopted the low-fat diet in 1980, giving rise to the American diet. This was low in fat and had loads of sugar and processed grains (which quickly changes to sugar in the body)
- With this in the picture, CVD was directly linked to fat consumption and lipid profiles
- Pharma industries caught on the opportunity and people with high TGs and cholesterol (because of high consumption) were put on cholesterol-lowering drugs that had to be taken for a lifetime
- The patient never got treated because they avoided thinking of it as the culprit
- The processing industry lapped up the recommendations—sold 'fat-free' food products with huge amounts of salt, sugar, simple

carbohydrates and unhealthy colours, flavours, and additives

- Heart disease remained the number one killer even though we stopped eating ghee and globally low-fat products were flying off the shelves
- In the 2000s the narratives started to change— new guidelines for diets were released and the terms 'healthy fat' started to pop up in nutrition articles
- As a long-term effect, fresh guidelines for total and maximum sugar consumption were issued and products had to specify the net sugar contents on the food label

Most people may not have heard of metabolic syndrome, but that is likely to change. Once known mysteriously as Syndrome X, the condition, a precursor to heart disease and type 2 diabetes, is about to be transformed into a household name by the pharmaceutical industry and its partners in the medical profession.

Packaged Foods and Nutrition: An Indian Perspective

According to a 2017 study aimed at evaluating the healthiness of the Indian packaged food and beverage supply, India's 11 largest food and beverage companies scored low on the overall mean healthiness of products.

Most fast-foods, canned, boxed, and packaged foods undergo a series of processing and every series strips the foods of some nutrients. Food processing constitutes a number of different procedures including heating, refining, preserving, and storing among others.

The Ministry of Food Processing of India (MOSPI) segregates the food processing industry into the following segments:

- Dairy, fruits and vegetable processing
- Grain processing
- Meat and poultry processing
- Fisheries
- Consumer foods such as packaged foods, beverages and packaged drinking water

Effect of processing and storage of food

There are two types of vitamins: fat-soluble and water-soluble. Fat-soluble vitamins are more stable and are less affected by processing while water-soluble vitamins are more unstable.

The most unstable vitamins include:
- Thiamine
- Folate
- Vitamin C

More stable vitamins include:

- Vitamin K
- Niacin (vitamin B3)
- Vitamin D
- Biotin (vitamin B7)
- Pantothenic acid (vitamin B5)

Processes affecting food nutrient content

Milling

Cereals like wheat lose their dietary fibre, B-group vitamins, photochemical, and some minerals during the removal of stringy husks. That is the reason white bread is considered less healthful than wholemeal varieties, even if they are artificially fortified with the lost nutrients.

Blanching

Before the process of canning or freezing, the food is subjected to quick heating with steam or water. This process of blanching strips the food of the soluble vitamins including B-complex and vitamin C.

Canning

The cans containing processed food are heated to kill any dangerous micro-organisms. While the process helps increase the shelf life of food, it may affect the food item's taste and texture.

Dehydrating

Drying out foods including fruits may destroy their vitamin C content. In addition, dehydration may also enhance the energy density of food, which is associated with weight gain.

Typical Maximum Nutrient Losses (as compared to raw food)

Vitamins	Freeze	Dry	Cook	Cook+ Drain	Reheat
Vitamin A	5%	50%	25%	35%	10%
Retinol Activity Equivalent	5%	50%	25%	35%	10%
Alpha Carotene	5%	50%	25%	35%	10%
Beta Carotene	5%	50%	25%	35%	10%
Beta Cryptoxanthin	5%	50%	25%	35%	10%
Lycopene	5%	50%	25%	35%	10%
Lutein+ Zeaxanthin	5%	50%	25%	35%	10%
Vitamin C	30%	80%	50%	75%	50%
Thiamin	5%	30%	55%	70%	40%
Riboflavin	0%	10%	25%	45%	5%
Niacin	0%	10%	40%	55%	5%
Vitamin B6	0%	10%	50%	65%	45%
Folate	5%	50%	70%	75%	30%

Food Folate	5%	50%	70%	75%	30%
Folic Acid	5%	50%	70%	75%	30%
Vitamin B12	0%	0%	45%	50%	45%
Minerals	**Freeze**	**Dry**	**Cook**	**Cook+ Drain**	**Reheat**
Calcium	5%	0%	20%	25%	0%
Iron	0%	0%	35%	40%	0%
Magnesium	0%	0%	25%	40%	0%
Phosphorus	0%	0%	25%	35%	0%
Potassium	10%	0%	30%	70%	0%
Sodium	0%	0%	25%	55%	0%
Zinc	0%	0%	25%	25%	0%
Copper	10%	0%	40%	45%	0%

Packaging material

Food business operators have a multitude of options when it comes to primary packaging. They pick their preferences on the basis of a number of criteria including product quality, customer requirements, and safety and inherent costs. Broadly, primary packaging involves four major material options: paper and board, glass, metals, and plastics.

Paper and board

Paper-based packaging's advantage to other materials is in relation to its environmental aspect because it is produced from sustainable and renewable resources. It is estimated that over 50% of the paper and paperboard used for packaging finds its application in the food industry. Listed below are some examples of paper- and paperboard-based packaging:

- Infusible tissues and packaging papers including tea and coffee bags, sugar and flour bags, sachets and pouches
- Fibre drums
- Diaphragms (membranes) and cap liners (sealing wads)
- Paper-based tubes, tubs, and composite containers
- Moulded pulp containers
- Liquid packaging

Natural products like paper-based material also are biodegradable and compost well without polluting the soil or watercourses and are suitable for recycling. Whilst paper-board is approved for packaging many food products, but the material alone is permeable to water, aqueous solutions, water vapour and fatty substances (except grease-resistant paper grades), and gases including oxygen, nitrogen, and carbon dioxide. Therefore, paper-board packaging is coated or laminated with leakage-proof material like polyethylene terephthalate (PET or PETE), polyethylene (PE), polypropylene (PP), and ethylene vinyl alcohol (EVOH) as well as aluminium foil, wax, among others to make them impermeable.

Glass

Glass is actually a super-cooled liquid. While it is fragile to handle, it is an ideal storage material for most of the food products without the risk of contamination. However, it is advised not to use coloured glass other than brown or green as coloured glasses cannot be recycled as the pigments may cause contamination. Glass finds its wide application for packaging chemicals, pharmaceuticals, food, beverages, cosmetics, and other materials.

Plastics

The use of plastics in food packaging gained momentum at the beginning of the 1990s, amounting to 28% of the market share. Today, a multitude of plastics are available. While some are sourced from natural materials, modern plastics produced from chemicals obtained from crude oil are also available. Today, the form of plastic most widely used for packaging is polyethylene.

While plastics are lighter than other packaging material including glass and metal, they have an edge over paper and boards due to their water and moisture resistant properties. However, being a non-degradable material, plastic is not good for the ecosystem. Moreover, the silver lining used inside the packages may lead to many health issues. That's the reason many states in India have banned the use of plastics for packaging and storage.

Metal

Metal, in the form of cans, is preferred for storing and packaging drinks and food products. Aluminium is extensively used in the packaging industry, thanks to its lightweight form, impermeability, thermal conduction, flexibility, and recyclability. However, studies have cited some harmful effects of using aluminium for packaging. Researchers suggest a possible link between aluminium levels in brain and Alzheimer's disease. The presence of aluminium in the human brain may be attributed to the aluminium packaging, which is used to store a number of food products, especially cans used for carbonated and non-carbonated beverages, like colas and fruit drinks.

Aluminium is used primarily in the following forms in the packaged food industry:

- **Aluminium Foils:** Aluminium foils find their extensive application in the packaging of fresh and processed poultry, fish, and meat. In addition, aluminium foils are also used in households for packaging breads, rotis and other food products.
- **Preserved foods:** Aluminium packages including pouches, foiled containers and laminated cartons have replaced traditionally used glass jars and metal cans as a preferred storage and packaging media for storing seasonal foodstuffs such as pickles, squashes and other similar stuff.
- **Dry and dehydrated foods:** Aluminium foils are

used to package dry and dehydrated foods for their ability to prevent the ingress of moisture while retaining the subtle flavours. Sachets made up of aluminium foils are widely used to pack dried food products, including milk and soup powders, vegetables, herbs and spices, and instant beverages.

• **Aluminium beverage cans:** The aluminium cans are extensively used to pack and store popular beverages such as carbonated and still soft drinks, beers, and lagers.

Advantages and Disadvantages of Major Food Packaging Material

Material	Rewards	Risks
Paper and board	• Manufactured from sustainable and renewable resources • Biodegradable and eco-friendly	• Paper-board alone is permeable to water, aqueous solutions, water vapour and fatty substances and gases
Glass	• Made from natural materials such as soda ash, sand, limestone, glass • The only packaging material recommended by the FDA as fully safe • Does not interfere with the quality of food products	• Bulkier and fragile • Risk of injury in case of breakage

Material	Rewards	Risks
Plastics	• Flexible and adaptable form of packaging • Extremely light-weight storage option • Can withstand extreme environments	• Plastic can melt, posing a risk of chemicals leaking into the food • BPA present in plastics can affect brain function, prostate function, and hormone levels
Aluminium	• Strong and durable • Light in weight • An excellent conductor of heat • Impermeable to light, gases, and liquids • Highly malleable and ductile	• Seepage of harmful chemicals from aluminium packaging is associated with various diseases including dementia, Alzheimer's, and cancer

Weighing down the risk vs reward ratio

Risk   Paperboard Packaging   Reward

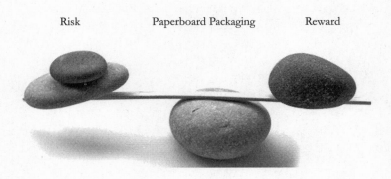

Risk Management:

It is definitely safer than aluminium and plastics. However, avoid using paperboard packaging that comes insulated with silver lining or aluminium foils. It can result in seeping of harmful chemicals in the food, thereby increasing the risk of mental health problems and some cancers.

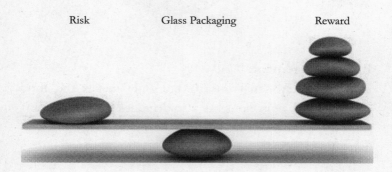

Risk Management:

On any day, glass is the safest packaging medium compared to other packaging material used for food. Taking adequate precautionary measures can help deal with associated risks. It may be costlier than plastic but safe for health.

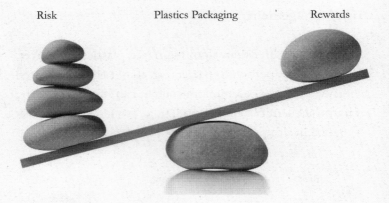

Risk   Plastics Packaging   Rewards

Risk Management:
It is extremely dangerous. It not only makes the food packaged in it poisonous but also degrades the eco-system.

Bottom line: Avoid to the core. It is already banned in many Indian states.

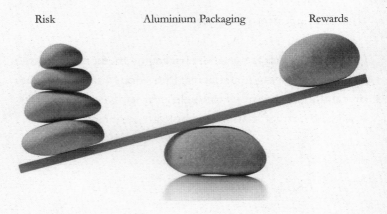

Risk   Aluminium Packaging   Rewards

Risk Management		
Facts in Favour	Concerns	Alternatives
Aluminium packaging is a trusted and a consistently used packaging material.	• Researchers cite a direct correlation between aluminium levels in the brain and Alzheimer's disease. • The cans used for carbonated and non-carbonated beverages, like colas and fruit drinks, leak significant amounts of aluminium into the beverage. • Apart from Alzheimer's disease, aluminium uptake is also linked to long-term and irreversible Parkinson's disease and dementia.	• One main alternative to aluminium packaging would be glass. • Glass is endlessly recyclable, with no significant risk of leakage into food items. • In addition, steel packaging is also safe compared to aluminium.

Get Back to Your Kitchens

Let me conclude the discussion with this: get back to your kitchens. Cook your meals and eat them fresh. According to a study, cooking dinner at home was found to induce healthy dietary patterns. The study suggested that consumption of daily servings of fresh produce increased by 3% for each additional trip to a grocery store, by 76% for shopping at a farmer's market, and by 38% for preparing food at home.

These findings are significant in the view that consumption of fruit and vegetable is known to promote health while minimizing the risk of diseases including hypertension, CVD, type 2 diabetes, osteoporosis, and cancer, as fruits and vegetables supply rich amounts of vital nutrients including potassium, minerals, vitamins, folate, and dietary fibre.

According to a study presented at the American Public Health Association's Annual Meeting in New Orleans, Louisiana, on November 17, 2014, which also appeared online in the journal *Public Health Nutrition*, people who frequently cook meals at home eat healthier and consume fewer calories than those who cook less.

"When people cook most of their meals at home, they consume fewer carbohydrates, less sugar and less fat than those who cook less or not at all, even if they are not trying to lose weight," said Julia A Wolfson, MPP, a CLF-Lerner Fellow at the Johns Hopkins Center for a Livable Future and lead author of the study.

It was found that people who cooked dinner six to seven nights per week consumed less fat and sugar per day compared to those who cooked dinner zero to once per week.

Wolfson added that there may not be a one-size-fits-all solution to getting people to cook more. "Time and financial constraints are important barriers to healthy cooking and frequent cooking may not be feasible for everyone. But people who cook infrequently may benefit from cooking classes, menu preparation coaching, or even lessons in how to navigate the grocery store or read calorie counts on menus in restaurants"

Another study linked home-cooking to better health at less expense. The study appeared from the University of Washington Health Sciences/UW Medicine showed that people who cook at home more often have increased benefits of eating a healthier overall diet.

"By cooking more often at home, you have a better diet at no significant cost increase, while if you go out more, you have a less healthy diet at a higher cost," said Adam Drewnowski, Director of the UW Center for Public Health Nutrition.

What was surprising to Drewnowski was that the study showed there was no increase in costs for eating a healthier diet. Home-cooked meals were associated with diets lower in calories, sugar and fat, but not with higher monthly expenses for food.

Now that there are no second thoughts on the benefits of home-cooked over packaged foods, it the time you realize the importance of consuming home-cooked foods and consuming more fruits and vegetables than packaged food. And, that's why many governmental and non-governmental organizations across the world promote home cooking as a key component of strategies to tackle obesity and poor quality diets.

Eating packaged foods is an addiction, which only harms your health and well-being. Do yourself a favour, return to your kitchens. Cook your meals and prefer the traditional cooking techniques rather than using the microwave way of cooking.

ACKNOWLEDGEMENT

My journey from a nutritionist to an author would not be complete without the persistent support and guidance of my mentor, Dr Alok Chopra. I am obliged to him for helping me look at functional nutrition and health in a new light. He is responsible for instilling in me a fresh perspective towards healing and disease remission that is reflected in my day-to-day clinical practice.

I am thankful to my husband for his unconditional support and to my two daughters who continue to inspire me to continuously broaden my horizons.

Kudos to my editor, Pooja Dadwal, who left no stone unturned to ensure that the final manuscript was flawless as well as a delightful read!